BEAUTY RULES

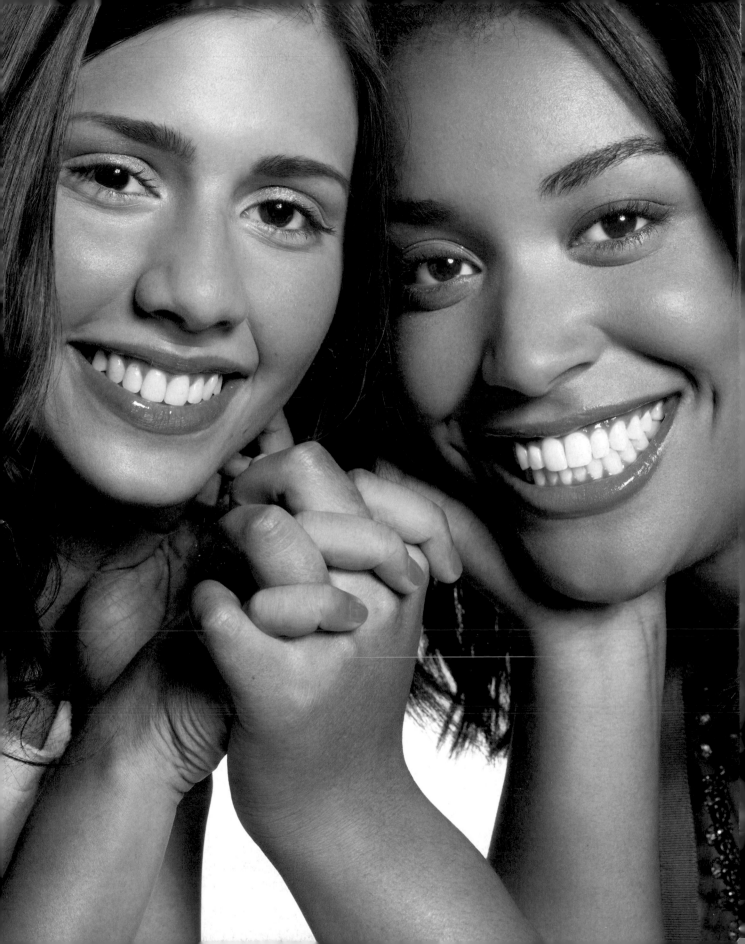

BEAUTY RULES

FABULOUS LOOKS, BEAUTY ESSENTIALS, AND LIFE LESSONS FOR
LOVING YOUR TEENS AND TWENTIES

BOBBI BROWN

WITH REBECCA PALEY
FOREWORD BY HILARY DUFF
PHOTOGRAPHS BY ONDREA BARBE AND BEN RITTER

CHRONICLE BOOKS

SAN FRANCISCO

I DEDICATE THIS BOOK TO MY SONS—DYLAN, DAKOTA, AND DUKE; MY NEPHEWS—JEREMY, TYLER, JAKE, ZACK, OWEN, AND NATE; MY NIECES—REBECCA, JESSICA, SAMANTHA, AND SYDNEY.

I LOVE YOU AND LOVE BEING AROUND YOU. I'LL CHOOSE TO BELIEVE YOU ARE ALWAYS LAUGHING WITH ME—NOT AT ME.

BOBBI

First Chronicle Books LLC paperback edition, published in 2014.

Copyright © 2010 by Bobbi Brown.
Cover photograph © 2013 by Ben Ritter.
All rights reserved. No part of this book may be reproduced in any form without written permission from the publisher.

ISBN 978-1-4521-1275-6

The Library of Congress has cataloged the original edition as follows:

Library of Congress Cataloging-in-Publication Data:
Brown, Bobbi.
Beauty rules : fabulous looks, beauty essentials, and life lessons for loving your teens and twenties / Bobbi Brown with Rebecca Paley; photographs by Ondrea Barbe and Ben Ritter.
p. cm.
Includes index.
ISBN 978-0-8118-7468-7
 1. Beauty, Personal. 2. Skin—Care and hygiene. I. Paley, Rebecca. II. Title.

RA778.B8784 2010
646.7'26—dc22

2009047126

Manufactured in China

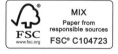

MIX
Paper from responsible sources
FSC® C104723
www.fsc.org

Designed by Sara Schneider

Portrait of Bobbi Brown on pages 7 and 12 and back cover courtesy of Henry Leutwyler

Compact photo on page 93 and brush photos on page 111 courtesy of Brian Hagiwara

Photograph of Coco Rocha on page 242 courtesy of Guy Aroch/trunkarchive.com

Barbie Doll is a registered trademark of Mattel, Inc. BlackBerry is a registered trademark of Research in Motion Ltd. Bobbi Brown's BBU Palette and Pot Rouge are registered trademarks of Bobbi Brown Professional Cosmetics, Inc. Bullfrog is a registered trademark of Oceanside Laboratories Corp. CamelBak is a registered trademark of CamelBak Products. Coke and Diet Coke are registered trademarks of the Coca-Cola Co. Cole Haan is a registered trademark of Cole Haan. Converse is a registered trademark of Converse, Inc. Coppertone is a registered trademark of Schering-Plough HealthCare Products, Inc. Council of Fashion Designers of America is a registered trademark of Council of Fashion Designers of America, Inc. Day-Glo is a registered trademark of Day-Glo Color Corp. Double RL and Ralph Lauren are registered trademarks of PRL USA Holdings, Inc. Girl Scouts is a registered trademark of Girl Scouts of the United States of America Corp. Gucci is a registered trademark of Gucci America, Inc. Italian Vogue and Vogue are registered trademarks of Advance Magazine Publishers, Inc. Izod is a registered trademark of the Phillips-Van Heusen Corp. J. Crew is a registered trademark of J. Crew International, Inc. Lilly Pulitzer is a registered trademark of Sugartown Worldwide, Inc. LPGA and Women's World Golf Rankings are registered trademarks of the Ladies Professional Golf Association. Lucky Charms is a registered trademark of General Mills, Inc. Neutrogena Active Sport is a registered trademark of the Neutrogena Corp. Photoshop is a registered trademark of Adobe Systems, Inc. Polo Ralph Lauren is a registered trademark of PRL USA Holdings, Inc. Prada is a registered trademark of Prada S.A. Corp. Proactiv is a registered trademark of Guthy-Renker Corp. Q-tips is a registered trademark of Unilever Supply Chain, Inc. Seventeen Magazine is a registered trademark of Hearst Communications, Inc. Tend Skin is a registered trademark of Tend Skin International, Inc. the Today show is a registered trademark of MSNBC Marks Trust. Tommy Hilfiger is a registered trademark of Tommy Hilfiger Licensing. Tory Burch is a registered trademark of River Light. US Open is a registered trademark of the United States Tennis Association, Inc. Walkers is a registered trademark of Walker's Shortbread Ltd.

10 9 8 7 6 5 4 3 2 1

Chronicle Books LLC
680 Second Street
San Francisco, California 94107
www.chroniclebooks.com

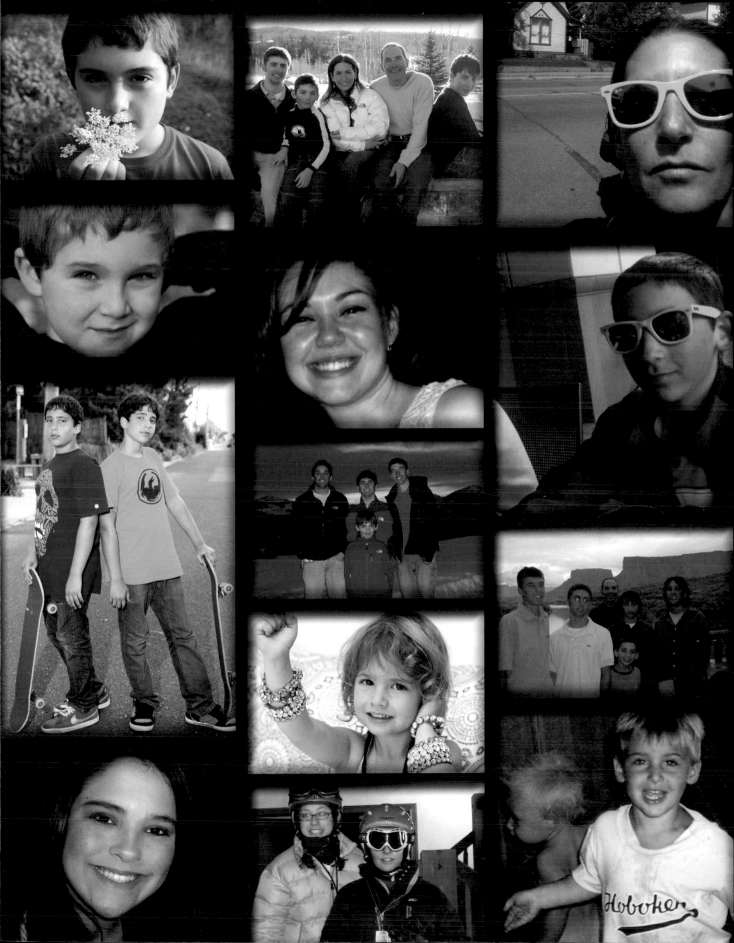

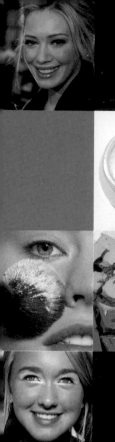

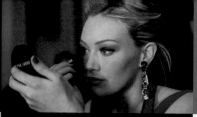

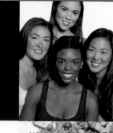

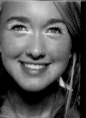

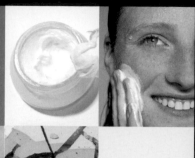

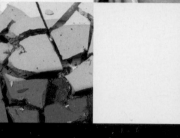

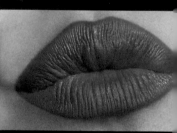

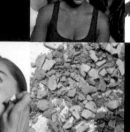

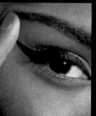

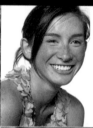

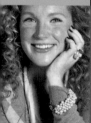

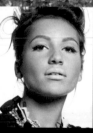

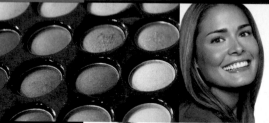

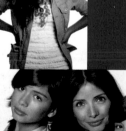

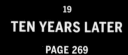

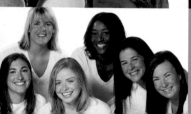

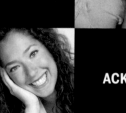

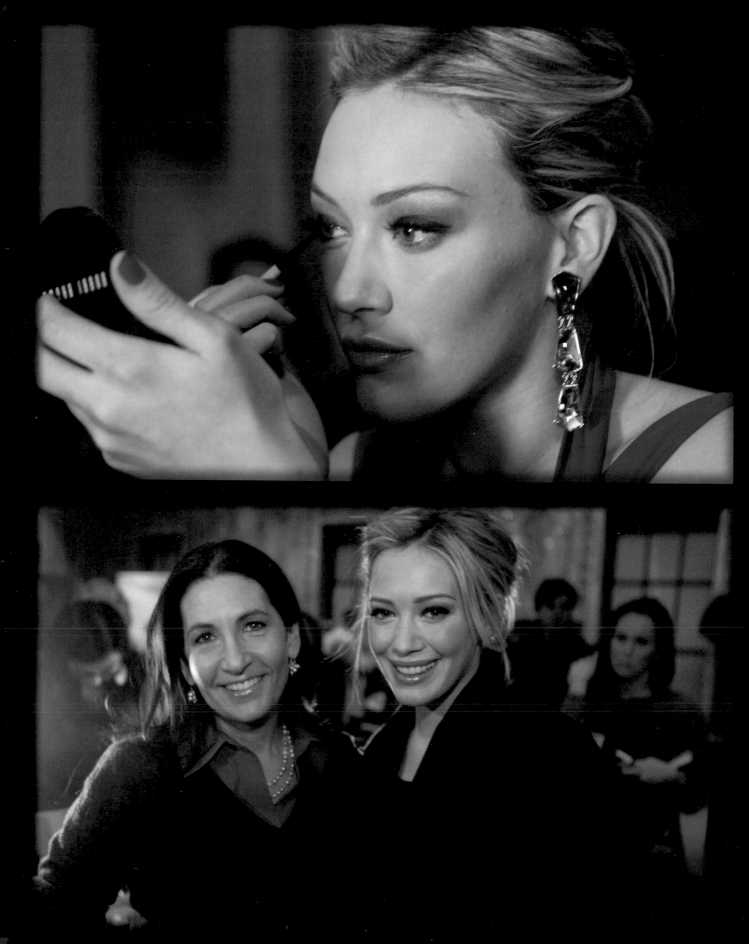

FOREWORD
I AM A WORK-IN-PROGRESS

At the early ages of 12 and 10, my older sister Haylie and I arrived in L.A. hoping to explore our creative talents and fulfill our dreams. From the very first day my mother was honest with us, explaining that we would face many new challenges and experiences; it was up to us to determine how they would influence our lives. Wisely, she advised us to embrace the positive, learn from the negative, and steer clear of the destructive. I quickly learned that there was to be no place for greed and jealousy and I should compete only with myself to do better. The path was simple: Despite what others may say or do, always stay true to yourself and your family.

With our fair share of mistakes and failures and eventually our cherished first successes, we each found our own niches in the entertainment industry. Seemingly overnight, I went from the unknown Texas "tomboy in a tutu" to Lizzie McGuire, the girl on television who everyone knew and liked just for being herself. Greater perseverance and more good fortune led to success in movies and music; creating fashion, home, and beauty brands; and taking on a meaningful role in charitable causes. Through everything, I have had to learn about patience and humility and, most important, to develop a very good sense of humor. I am still a work-in-progress.

Evolving from a girl to a young woman in a very public way, I learned very quickly that I could not project a positive public persona until I really became aware of my own unique self—both fabulous and flawed. We all have a list of things about our appearance and character that we would like to change or improve. At times I wish I were taller or that my shoulders were less broad—physical attributes I cannot change. That has never stopped me from loving fashion or dressing to express myself. I believe that those self-perceived imperfections have challenged my personal character and freed me to create my own special look. When we feel that all eyes are upon on us, it is often difficult to take chances in expressing our individuality. But my advice is: Always take that chance. Carry yourself with confidence; if you learn to like what you see in the mirror, others will too. It's worth the risk!

Years before my sister and I were born, my mother started to work as a makeup artist, a career that helped her find her independence as a young woman and allowed her to reach out to others to make a difference in their lives. Perhaps that's why I have a fondness for makeup and talented makeup artists such as Bobbi Brown. Bobbi is legendary as a creative force in the cosmetics industry. She is an innovator, entrepreneur, teacher, and celebrated author. As a philanthropist she has shared her time, energy, and money to help teens from the Jane Addams High School for Academic Careers in the Bronx prepare to realize their full potential and she has helped disadvantaged women enrolled in the Dress for Success program regain their self-worth as they prepare to reenter the workforce. Giving is beautiful!

I first met Bobbi when she did my makeup for The Heart Truth's Red Dress Collection fashion show, an annual New York Fashion Week event in which celebrities model red dresses designed by top designers to raise awareness of women's heart health. With make-up, as in life, there is an art to accentuating natural beauty and lovingly minimizing flaws. Because of Bobbi, each one of us walked the catwalk radiating beauty and confidence that day.

Beauty is defined in so many ways. Like Bobbi, I find it hard to believe that physical beauty can thrive without cultivating inner beauty. In everything that she says and does, Bobbi reminds us to value the natural beauty of all women. She has empowered us as teens and women alike to celebrate our similarities and yet still be confident to embrace our differences in expressing our own unique selves. Finding out all the ways that we are beautiful beings is a worthy cause.

As you read Bobbi's book, keep in mind: We are all beautiful works-in-progress.

Love yourself.

Hilary Duff

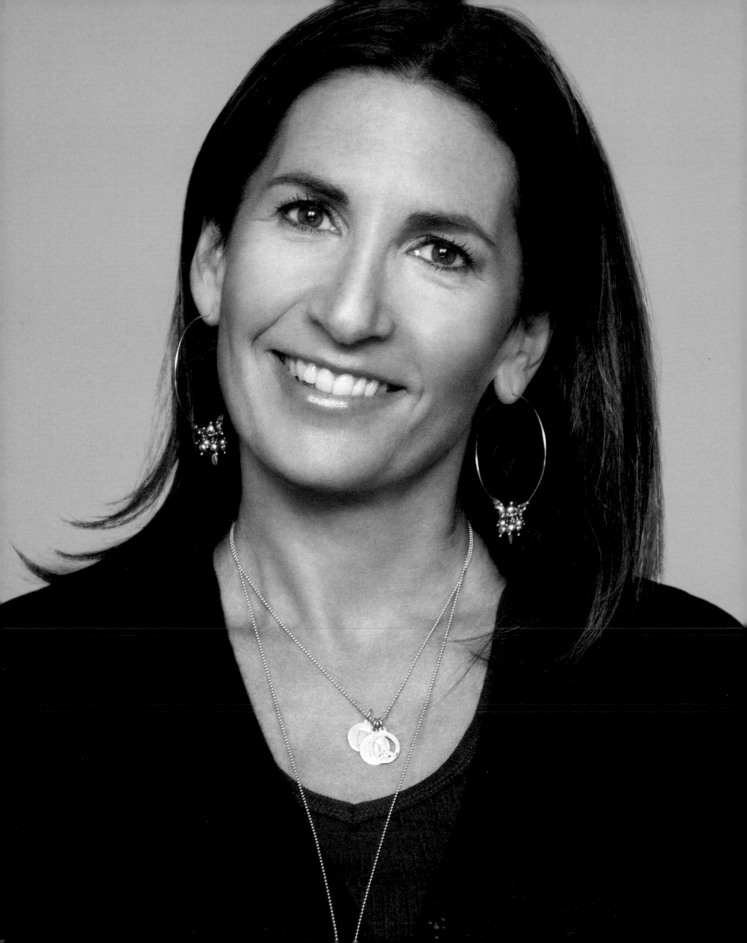

1

BOBBI BARES ALL

I haven't always been the confident woman I am today. Part of my job is making the world's most beautiful people and biggest celebrities look their best for photo shoots, red carpet events, and fashion shows. If I didn't believe in me, they wouldn't believe in me. I'm also a bit naive and never think that I can't do something. I'm a business-woman running a big company that sells beauty products all over the world. I've written best-selling books and made countless television appearances. And I have to deal with plenty of powerful people, including movie stars, top photographers, and even a few American presidents. Oh, and did I mention I live in a house filled with men (my husband and three sons)? If I weren't strong and self-assured, I'd never make it through my day.

But I haven't always been that way. Far from it. I was a bit inse-cure growing up. All I ever wanted to be when I was a teen was tall, blond, blue-eyed, flat-chested, and long-legged. And I am totally the opposite of all those things. But that style was really in when I was a teen. So even though I was the shortest girl in class, with dark brown hair and eyes, and a big chest, that unattainable blond chick in my head was my ideal. Whenever I looked in the mirror, I felt disappointment at what I saw. For a long time, I just didn't think I was pretty.

Because I wasn't satisfied with my image, I spent a lot of time trying to figure out my look. I went from parting my waist-length hair down the middle and wearing chunky turquoise jewelry to dressing the part of an '80s Madonna-wannabe—and many unmentionable looks in between. I'm a creative person, and trying out different things turned out to be a lot of fun. Throughout the evolution of my style, I always loved playing with makeup. Experimenting with bronzers, eyeliners, shadow, and lipstick meant transforming myself, and, of course, being prettier.

Makeup ended up being the way I found myself. It took me from a normal high school kid to a household name. Not that it happened overnight. The same determination I applied to figuring out my style I applied to launching my career—from designing my own "makeup" major in college to dealing with rejection as a beginning professional.

I love sharing what I've learned in my transformation—both personal and professional—with the countless young women I meet. A lot of them are confused about what to do with their own appearances. They want to feel and look better, but they don't know where to begin. I'm here to tell you that there's so much you can do to improve your looks. A great haircut, the right clothes, a kick-your-butt workout, a beautiful blush—small steps make a big difference. I now know which clothes work with my body and make me feel comfortable. I have my trusty black stretchy dress that looks great with sneakers during the day or with heels and big earrings at night. And I have denim down to a science. I also have a simple skin-care routine, quick makeup application, and a cut that's right for my hair. The important part is that I have figured out what works for *me*.

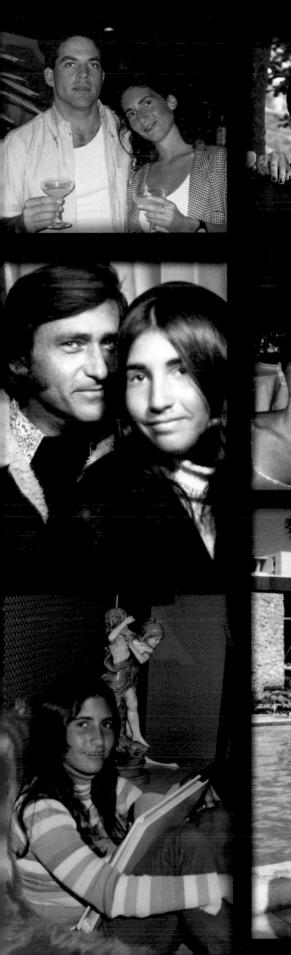
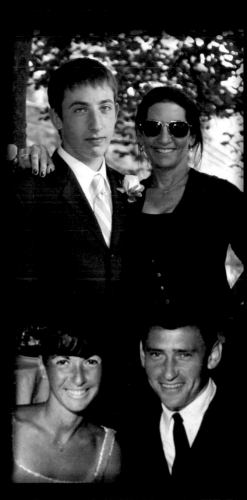
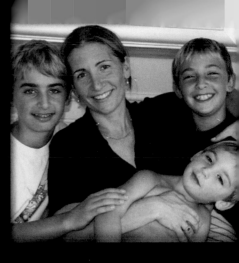
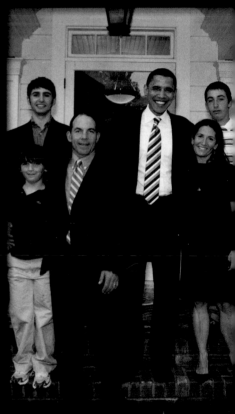
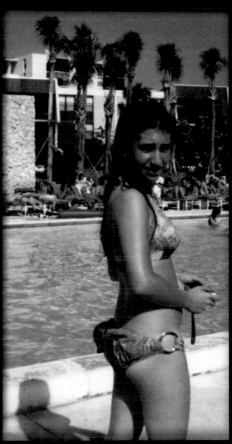
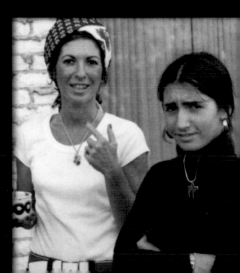

BOBBI'S BASIC LIFE RULES

Being happy is the best beauty tip I have. Nothing looks better than a big smile. Everyone has ups and downs, but it's important to stay focused on what makes you feel good. These rules have never failed.

RULE NUMBER 1: BE NICE
I'M NOT KIDDING.

This is rule Number One and it's not negotiable. You must be kind whether you are talking to a waiter, a teacher, or your mother (okay, you can be a little bit rude to your family members once in a while).

THE MORE YOU GIVE TO OTHERS, THE MORE YOU GET.

RULE NUMBER THREE: TAKE RISKS

I came to New York to become a makeup artist without knowing anyone or anything. So I picked up the phone book and cold-called anyone who was listed under makeup or modeling.

IT WAS CRAZY, BUT THAT'S HOW I BEGAN MY CAREER.

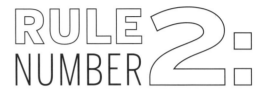

RULE NUMBER 2: TELL THE TRUTH

IT'S NOT JUST THE RIGHT THING TO DO. HONESTY ALSO SAVES TIME. LIFE IS JUST SIMPLER AND EASIER WHEN YOU ARE TRUTHFUL WITH OTHERS, AND WITH YOURSELF.

RULE NO. 4: NEVER GIVE UP

WHEN I STARTED WORKING IN MAKEUP I HAD NO EXPERIENCE. A LOT OF TIMES I HAD TO WORK FOR FREE TO PROVE MYSELF, AND SOMETIMES PEOPLE WOULDN'T EVEN LET ME DO THAT.

EVEN THOUGH I HAD REALLY DISCOURAGING DAYS, I NEVER LET NO BECOME THE FINAL ANSWER.

RULE NUMBER FIVE:

BE ON TIME

No one likes to be kept waiting. But if you are going to be more than five minutes late—call!

RULE NO. 7: CARE ABOUT SOMETHING

SPORTS. MUSIC. POLITICS.

ANYTHING YOU LIKE.
GET INVOLVED AND GET ACTIVE.

RULE NUMBER NINE:

WORK HARD

START AT THE BOTTOM AND LEARN ALL YOU CAN. BE STRONG. DON'T GET UPSET WHEN THINGS DON'T COME TO YOU RIGHT AWAY.

RULE NUMBER 6: BE OPEN!!!

While I was doing an in-store appearance, an older lady asked me for tips to make her lipstick last. I took time to give her my best advice, after which the lady said she thought I would be great on the *Today* show. I told her that was a big dream of mine. Turns out the little red-haired woman was the grandmother of the *Today* show's executive producer. That meeting helped me become the show's guest beauty editor.

RULE NUMBER EIGHT: GIVE BACK

THERE ARE SO MANY WAYS TO MAKE THIS WORLD A BETTER PLACE, WHETHER IT IS HELPING THE ENVIRONMENT, PEOPLE IN YOUR COMMUNITY, OR PLACES HALFWAY ACROSS THE GLOBE.

FIND A CAUSE THAT'S MEANINGFUL TO YOU AND MAKE IT YOUR OWN.

RULE NUMBER TEN:

LOOK PEOPLE IN THE EYE: IT SHOWS CONFIDENCE.

RULE NUMBER ELEVEN: DREAM BIG

YOU NEVER KNOW . . .

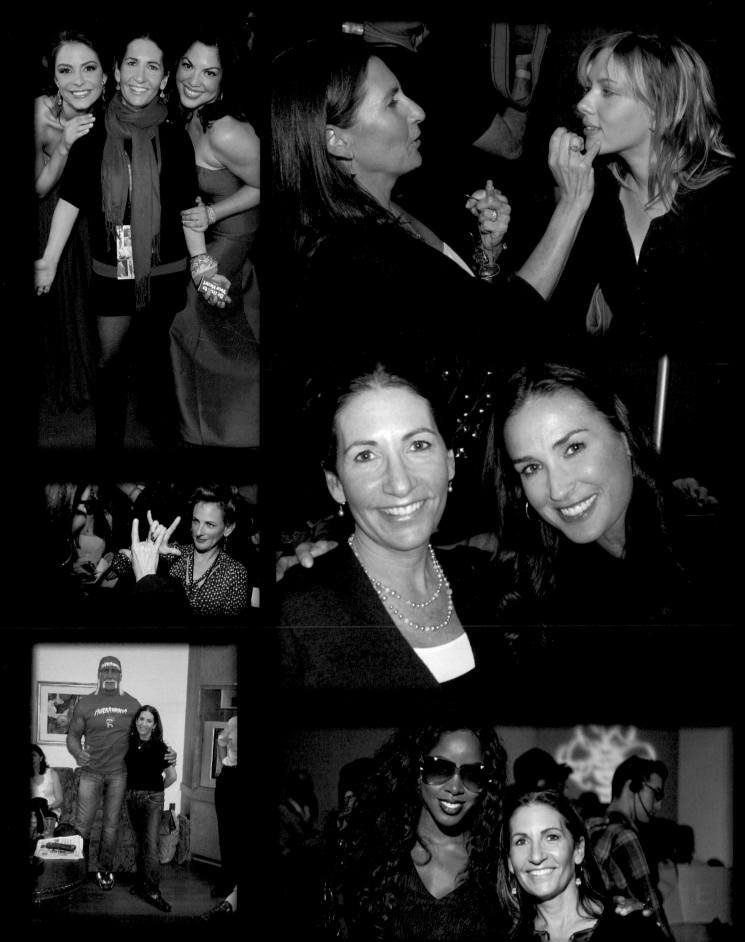

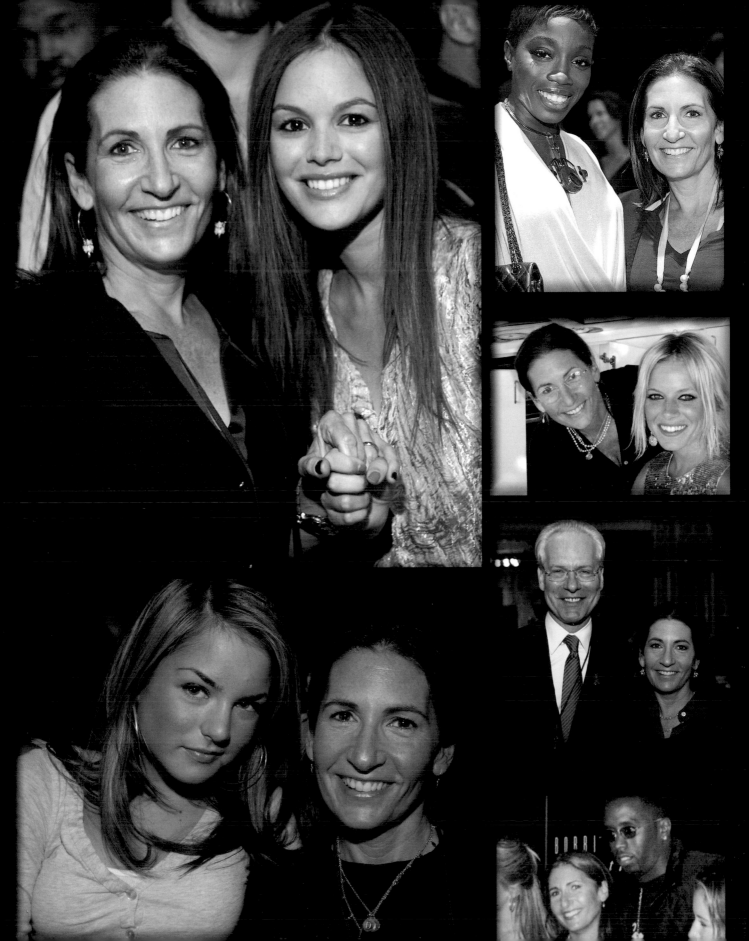

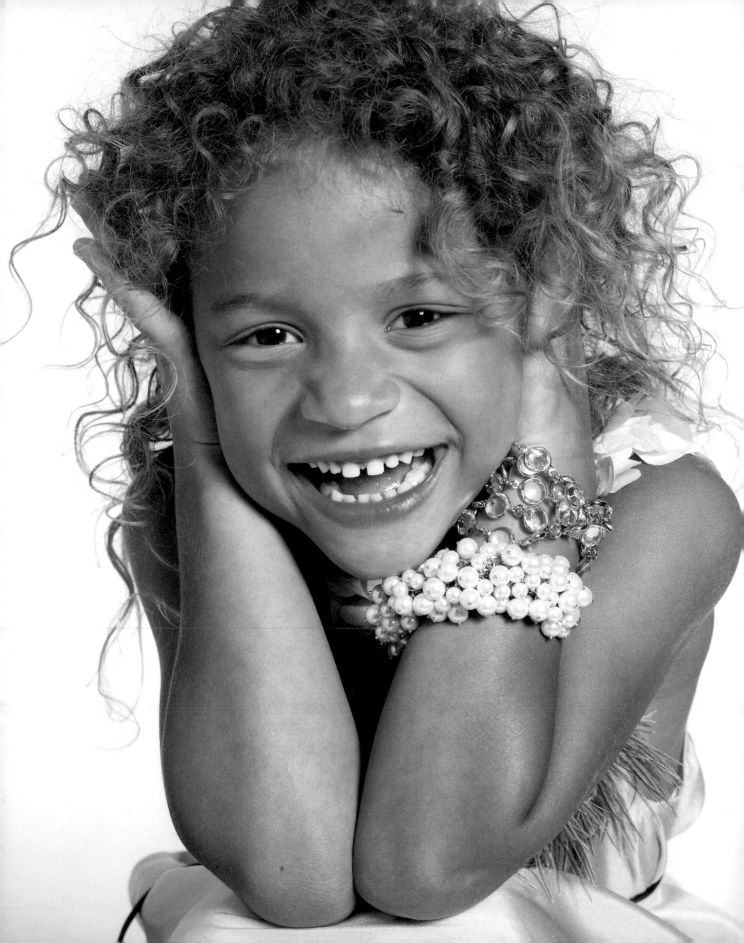

2

BEAUTY BEGINS

My love for makeup began by watching my mother put hers on before she went out at night. I sat fascinated as she applied cream bronzer, eye shadow, mascara, blush, and lipstick. I couldn't imagine a more glamorous and grown-up activity. And I couldn't wait to get my hands on all her stuff (which she let me do, long before she let me wear makeup out). Most little girls begin their love affair with makeup much the same way: by observing a sister, cousin, or mother and then later imitating these older role models.

All girls love to play with makeup. Lipstick, nail polish, and blush are pretty—just like sparkles, rhinestones, her mama's pearls, and, of course, the color pink.

But when are you old enough to get started really wearing makeup? Well, a lot of that depends on you (and, I guess, your parents). Some girls will run out to buy lip gloss the minute they collect the money from their first allowance, while others don't get interested until they're in high school. Only you can decide when you're ready to start playing with makeup seriously.

A GIRL'S NEVER TOO YOUNG TO LOVE BLING.

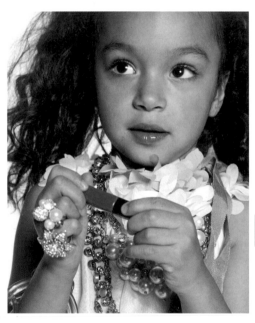 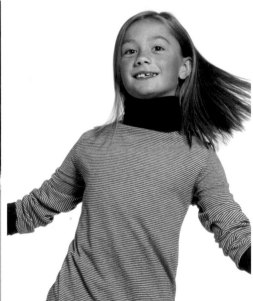 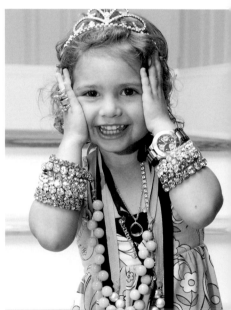

All girls, no matter how old they are, love to play with makeup and to dress up. It's just part of our DNA. Whether layering on lip gloss or jewels, have a good time experimenting with your look. There are no rules when it comes to fun.

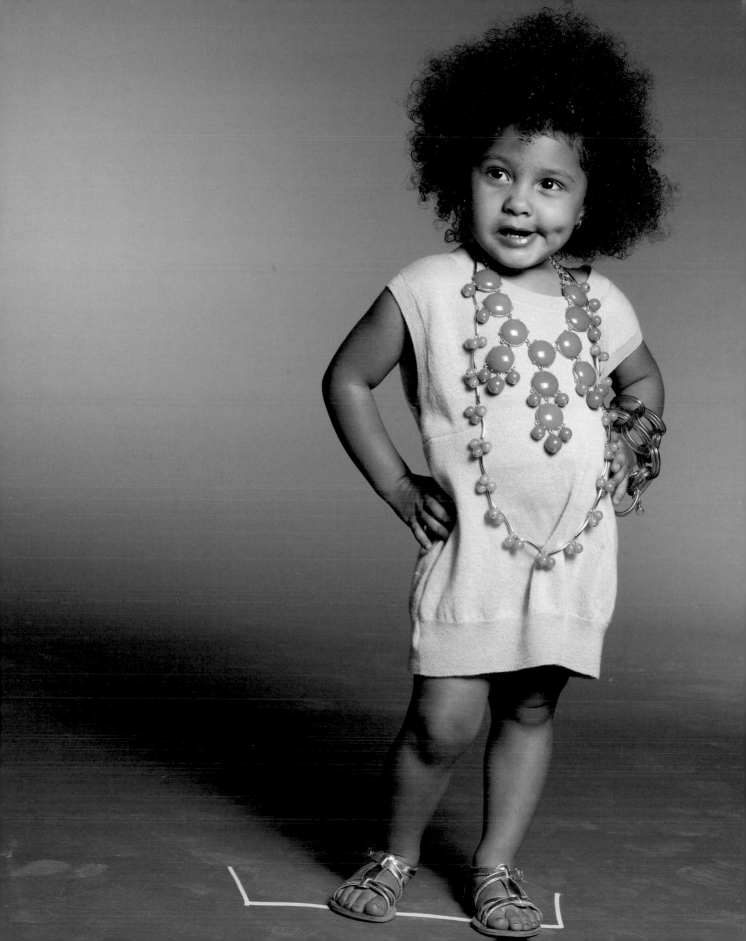

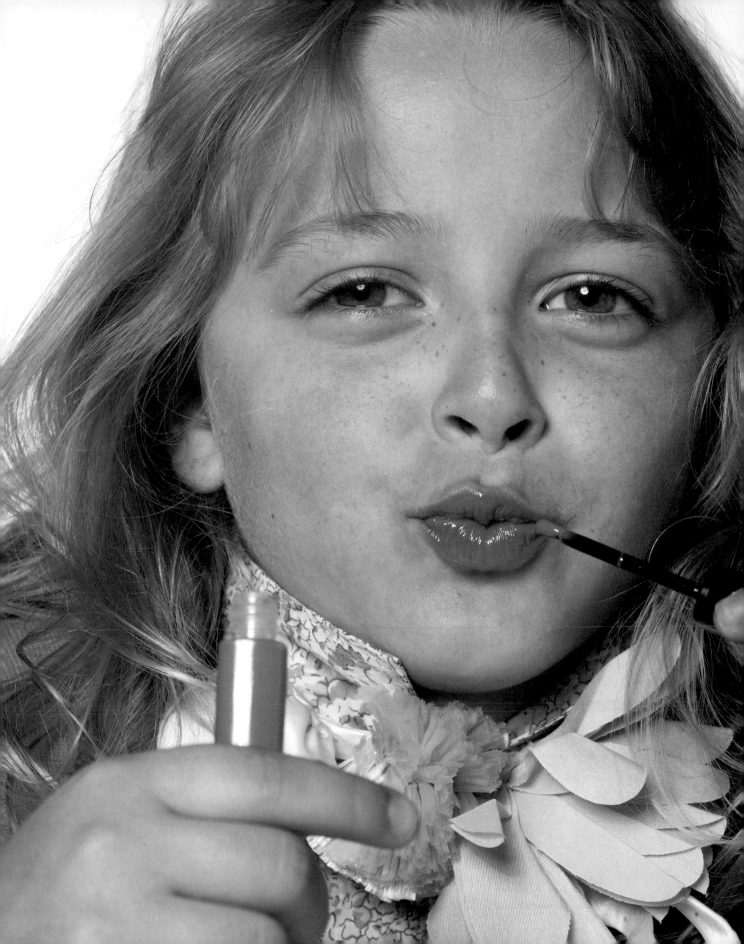

beauty on your time

Makeup is one thing, but what about eating well, exercising, wearing braces, and other stuff you might be starting to think about now that you're growing up? Here's my advice on when it might be right for you to add some of these elements to your own beauty routine. These are just general guidelines. Remember, everyone is different, so respect your own rhythms and interests.

EATING WELL

WHEN TO GET STARTED: Right away. It's never too early. I can't stress this enough. Eating fresh fruits and veggies, whole grains, dairy, and lean protein is one of the most important things you can do to look beautiful. I think it makes skin look better, and it definitely is the source for shiny hair and strong teeth and bones. Plus, it gives you the energy boost you need to get through your busy day (for more on good eating, see page 48). You may not make the decisions when it comes to food shopping at home or what they serve at school, but you have some say. Skip the soda and drink water instead. Head out to the grocery store with your parents once in a while. Take an interest in what goes into your body.

WHY DELAY: There's no reason. Now, I'm not talking about diets here. Please don't get confused. You are still growing and need all the nutrients you can get. If you are overweight, see a doctor or nutritionist who can guide you safely through a weight-loss program. Otherwise, skip the diets. And enjoy your favorite foods like fries, chocolate, and pizza in moderation. Just make healthy eating the rule, not the exception.

EXERCISE

WHEN TO GET STARTED: I'm an exercise fanatic and think you should do something each day to get your blood pumping. But I know not everyone is as into sports as I am. Still, the more you exercise, the more energy you'll have.

WHY DELAY: No reason. You don't need to join a gym or spend a lot of money on sports equipment to exercise. Some of the simplest forms of exercise are the best for your body. One example is jumping rope, which many top athletes do as part of their workout routine. If that's too intense for you, grab a friend and go for a brisk walk. As long as you can feel your heart beating faster or you are a little out of breath, it's all good.

DEODORANT

WHEN TO GET STARTED: You should only start wearing deodorant when you need to—that means when you have body odor. Everyone's body works differently. You might find you only sweat when you are working out or during very hot weather. Then you only need to wear deodorant at those times. However, it's perfectly normal to sweat all the time and wear deodorant every day.

WHY DELAY: No reason. If you do start wearing deodorant, don't pull out your dad's stinky antiperspirant and start rolling it on. Talc-free baby powder is great to start with. When you are ready, shop for a product that's right for you. I prefer natural deodorants that you can find in health food stores because they don't have as many chemicals as the mass-market brands. Also, opt for deodorant, which neutralizes the odor, over antiperspirant, which blocks the sweat. If you find that you sweat a ton, then you can move to a more heavy-duty formula.

SUNSCREEN

WHEN TO GET STARTED: Doctors say that babies who are six months old should start wearing sunscreen. And your mother probably started slathering it on you around then. But now you're too old for her to remind you to protect your skin (well, almost). You know to load up on high SPF sunscreen at the beach, but sunscreen isn't just for the surf. Start wearing a light moisturizer with SPF on ordinary days when you'll be outside (for more on sunscreen, see page 39).

WHY DELAY: Don't! The earlier you start protecting your skin from the sun's harmful rays with sunscreen, the better it will look later on. You are also doing important work in preventing the real threat of skin cancer that comes from burns and over-exposure to the sun.

MAKEUP

WHEN TO GET STARTED: If you are dying to wear makeup, by twelve years old I think it's okay to start using a little bit. *A little bit.* That means mascara and a swipe of lip gloss. Anything more, like a little blush and some sparkle on the eye, is for dances and parties only. Save the smoky eyes for when you're older.

WHY DELAY: Basically, I think nine is way too early. Learn to appreciate your face the way it is, and enjoy that incredible skin! Concentrate on friends and fun. That can include playing around with lipstick, nail polish, and some blush at home with your pals.

HAIR REMOVAL

WHEN TO GET STARTED: This is more about your body hair than it is about age. Some girls get thick, coarse leg and underarm hair before they hit their teens, and some never get it (lucky them). If you've got thick body hair growing, I can understand why you would want to get rid of it. Shaving is the easiest, least painful way to get started, but there are a variety of hair-removal options (for more on hair removal, see page 43).

WHY DELAY: If your hair is light and fuzzy, my advice is to hold off. Shaving or waxing might seem interesting and sophisticated before you do it. Once you start, though, it's hard to stop because of the way the hair grows back. The novelty quickly wears off, and you are left with another chore in your schedule.

HAIR COLORING

WHEN TO GET STARTED: I'm not a huge fan of girls younger than teenagers coloring their hair. Hair envy is a fact of life, like the sun rising or your parents bugging you about your homework. For some reason, we always want what we don't have when it comes to our hair. If you want to experiment with a different hair color, get a product that washes out of your hair. Do a colorful strip or a lighter tone all over. If you don't like it, you'll be happy it isn't permanent.

WHY DELAY: If you have black hair, you'll never be a blond. It might work for Madonna, but for the rest of us mere mortals, you'll just make a mess of your hair. Depending on what kind of color you use, it can damage the hair. Plus, to do it right with a professional, in a salon—can cost a lot of money. Spend some time and energy making what you do have look great (for more on hair, see Chapter 10).

BRACES

WHEN TO GET STARTED: Most kids get braces between the ages of ten and fourteen, while the head and mouth are still growing and teeth are easier to straighten. There are so many different choices these days when it comes to braces, including invisible, removable, and straight-up wire. If you think you are ready for braces, talk to your parents about visiting an orthodontist, who can walk you through all your options.

WHY DELAY: Getting braces before you have all your adult teeth is considered risky because you don't know what they will do before they grow into your mouth. Braces are also very expensive and take responsibility and maturity on the part of the wearer. (You need to avoid certain foods, wear your night brace and rubber bands, and follow the dentist's directions for years until they come off. It will be worth it. I promise!) So don't get braces until you are willing to take them seriously. If you get them on and feel self-conscious, don't worry. Deal with dry lips often caused by braces with some pretty, sheer tinted lip gloss. Play up your other features with a light-sheen shimmer eye shadow and a touch of blush.

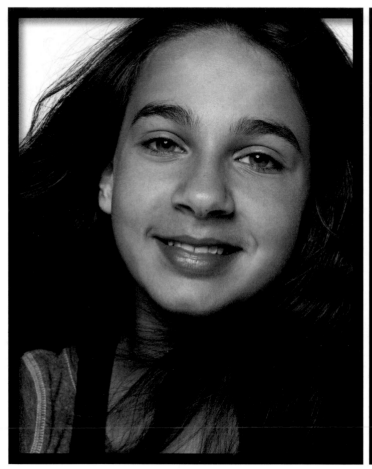 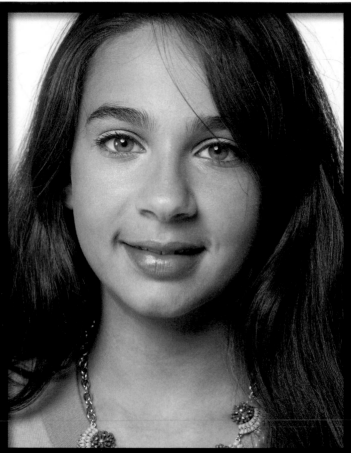

Hannah is naturally pretty without makeup, so it didn't take much to bring out her amazing features. A light sweep of sparkly shadow across her lids and a little eyeliner made her hazel eyes really pop. She didn't need any foundation. A pinkish, sheer lip gloss just pulls her whole gorgeous look together.

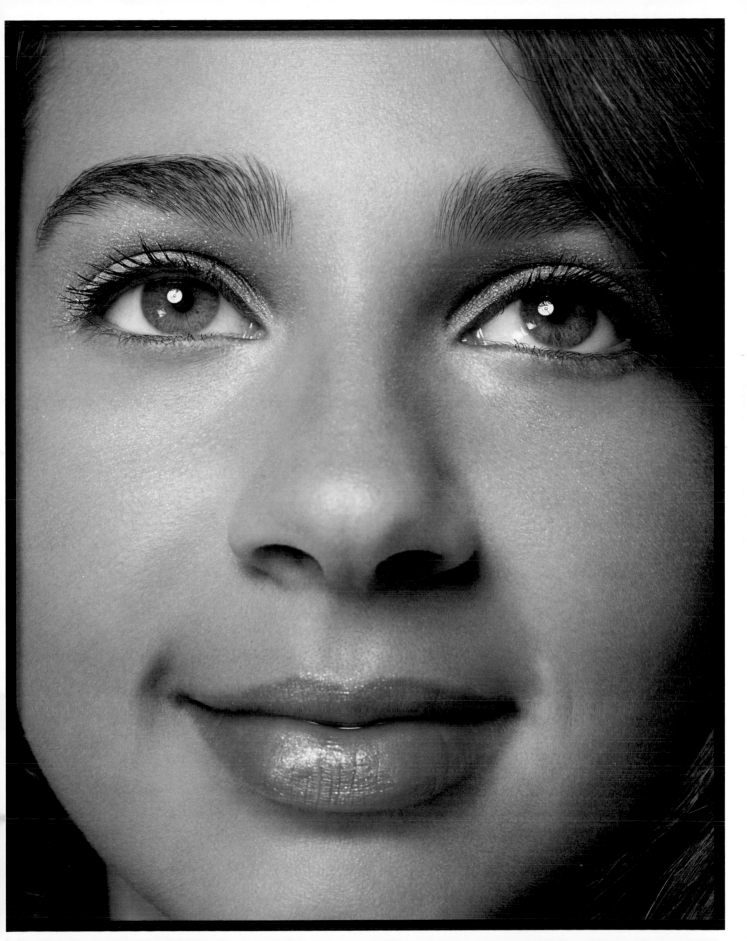

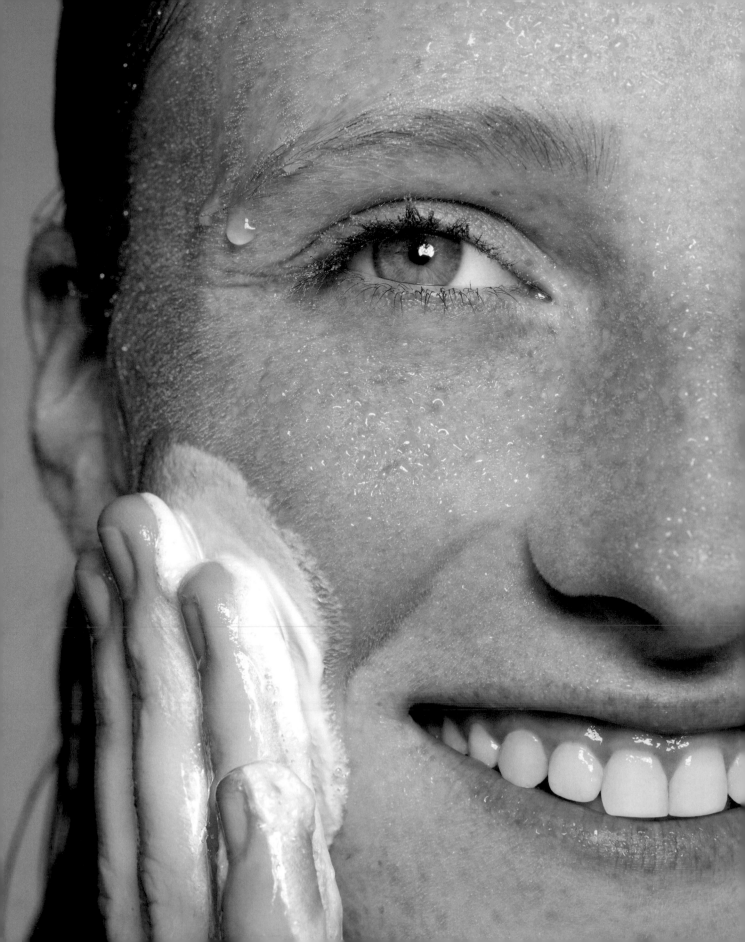

3

FEELING GOOD IN YOUR SKIN

I've always had pretty good skin. I'm lucky—I was born that way. Genes that you inherit from your parents do play a huge part in how your skin looks and how it ages. But the good news is that your DNA is not a life sentence. If you have problems with your skin—which most of us do—there are a lot of things you can do to improve it. The first step is taking responsibility. You'll probably have to try different products and routines before you find what's right for you. There is no perfect answer to anything. Even dermatologists sometimes have to try multiple solutions before they can fix a problem.

My secret to beautiful skin has a lot to do with what I put in my body. As a beauty expert and well-known health nut, I'm just as concerned about what I eat as the moisturizer I use (and believe me, I'm obsessed with moisturizer). Like any organ in your body, your skin will improve with good, clean, healthy foods. Luckily, even if you're having a bad skin day, month, or year, there are loads of makeup products to improve its appearance. But we'll get to that later. First, let's get your skin the most beautiful it can be.

the routine

"Routine" is not usually a word I like. When it comes to skin, however, I love it. Establishing good habits every day (yes, *every* day) is the most important thing you can do. If you skip washing your face after sweaty sports or a long day of wearing makeup, your pores can quickly clog and cause pimples.

the face

CLEAN IT

Pimples come from pores that are clogged with dead skin cells and have become infected. The basic idea behind clear skin is to keep your pores clean. This is more than just getting rid of dirt on your face. In fact, it's hard to wash inside the pore with regular soap. You need to use a product that gets deep inside the pore.

To find a cleanser that will get rid of dead skin cells, look for any of these ingredients in the label: salicylic acid, benzoyl peroxide (this has antibacterial properties but also bleaches clothing and skin), retinoids, glycolic acid, or lactic acid. All of these are doctor approved and come in regular, over-the-counter face washes.

Your skin type will determine the cleanser formula you should use.

OILY: Use an oil-free cleansing gel that doesn't dry out your skin.
NORMAL: Use a clear, foaming cleanser.
DRY: Use a non-foaming or creamy cleanser.

Don't tug on your skin when you are washing it. Use warm water and lightly apply the cleanser. If you want a bit of added exfoliation, use a washcloth while rinsing off.

A lot of girls who play sports find they break out if they don't instantly clean their face after working out. Bring a towel to your workout, soak it in water, and wipe off sweat from the face. Or you can look in the drugstore for face-cleansing pads that you can stash in your gym bag.

TONE IT

Toners are generally only useful if you have oily skin. But sometimes it feels so good to have that tingling sensation, which seems to scream *clean.* No matter what your skin type, don't use a straight alcohol toner. The product should not just strip your skin of oil, it should also deliver healing or antibacterial products, such as witch hazel or chamomile, to your skin.

MOISTURIZE IT

Moisturizer adds things to the skin to help it absorb and retain water after you've cleansed your face. That becomes more important as you get older, but it is necessary for anyone with dry skin. This may sound counterintuitive, but girls with oily skin need moisturizer, too. It's essential for delivering other things to the skin, such as vitamins or SPF. Look for oil-free moisturizers with sunscreen for everyday use in the morning and evening.

No matter what kind of skin you have, make sure your moisturizer is noncomedo-genic, which means it doesn't block pores. If you have dry skin, use a moisturizer with SPF during the daytime and cream (which has less water) at night.

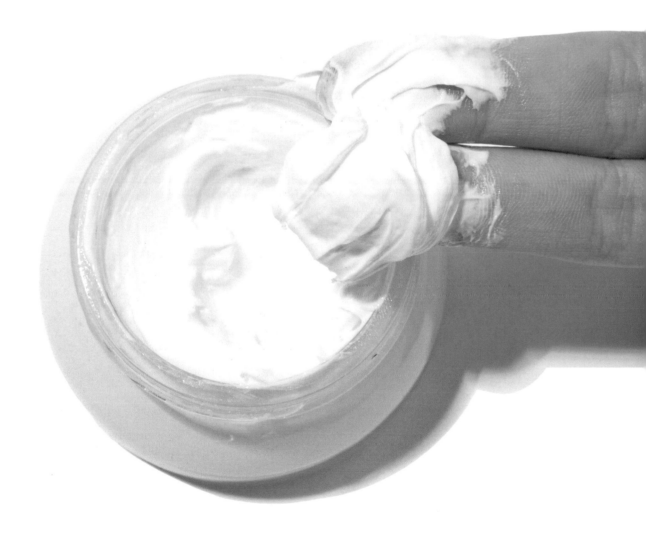

the body

CLEAN IT

Showering daily with the right soap is important for good hygiene. Everyone wants to be clean and smell good, but you also want to avoid drying out your skin.

When showering, keep the water at a warm temperature. I know super-hot water feels great, but it also dries skin. When soaping up, concentrate on areas that emit odor, such as underarms. You don't need to lather all over unless you are really dirty after camping or a massive workout.

If you get pimples on your back or chest, find a cleanser with salicylic acid that will exfoliate the pores. Anyone who wants smoother skin can use a grainy scrub product, loofah, or washcloth to physically exfoliate the skin and remove dead skin.

MOISTURIZE IT

Moisturizers for the body can be lotions, creams, or balms. The most effective time to apply is right after you've stepped out of the shower, when your skin is still damp. Another option if your skin is on the dry side: keep a spray bottle with baby or body oil in the shower. After you turn off the water, pat your skin dry with a towel. Then spray yourself with the oil.

Save the richest moisturizers for your hands and feet, which take a lot of abuse. If your feet crack in the winter (a common problem), rub the soles of your feet lightly for thirty seconds with a pumice stone in the shower to remove dead skin. Follow that immediately with a specially formulated foot cream that you can find in the drugstore or chemist aisle. Then put on a pair of gym socks to wear to bed or at least for a couple of hours. This will seal in the moisturizer to heal dry feet. You don't need to have super-dry feet to do this. Anyone who wants to pamper her feet once in a while should give it a try.

shop like a pro

When it comes to finding cleansers, deodorants, and moisturizers, don't just stick to your local drugstore or chemist or department store. I like to branch out to health food stores, where the products are all natural. I use a lot of organic and natural beauty supplies. Of course, the best all-natural experience comes from making your own beauty product. Make my favorite exfoliation scrub by combining kosher or rock salt or sugar and olive oil (just enough to make a paste out of the salt or sugar). Mix the ingredients together in a plastic container and scrub into the skin, then rinse. Be careful not to apply the salt scrub right after you've shaved, or it will burn.

zit zone

Conquering the pimple problem is not easy, especially when you're a teen. Acne is more common during the teenage years because of hormone changes that happen during that period. How you deal with a pimple depends on what kind it is, but in general you should try to avoid picking. The bacteria on your hands will get onto your face and just make the situation worse. Also, picking can lead to permanent scarring. Here's what you should do.

IF YOU HAVE MOSTLY WHITEHEADS: Use an over-the-counter medication with antibacterial properties. Benzoyl peroxide is a good option, because it also dries out the pimple. Whiteheads are tough to leave alone. If you get one you can't live with, take a washcloth and soak it with very hot water. Press the hot washcloth to the pimple gently and repeat until the pimple opens itself and drains.

IF YOU HAVE MOSTLY BLACKHEADS: Retinoids are great at exfoliating the pore, which is necessary for getting rid of blackheads or stopping them from occurring in the first place. If you have a lot of blackheads that aren't shrinking with a product, you might need to get them extracted with a facial. Go to someone who is medically trained and not just a place offering a soothing experience.

IF YOU HAVE DEEP-SEATED PIMPLES: These are the painful, red bumps that have no head at all. If you get this kind of acne, you should see a dermatologist because this acne is hard to treat with over-the-counter medicine and can lead to scarring. To find a dermatologist, ask your family doctor or friends to give you a referral. I'm not a fan of finding a doctor online or in the phone book. When you call a dermatologist, ask if the doctor is board certified and always ask the cost of an office visit.

disguising pimples

Makeup is a great ally when it comes to dealing with pimples, but you have to mask them the right way. Follow these simple steps to camouflage your zits.

STEP 1: Apply a little oil-free moisturizer on the pimple. This might seem counter-intuitive, but you want to smooth out the zit's rough surface before you disguise it.

STEP 2: After the skin has absorbed the moisturizer, use your finger or a small brush to cover the zit with foundation or blemish cover stick that matches your skin exactly. You can use a cream or stick foundation, but never use concealer lighter than your skin tone; concealer will only highlight your pimples.

STEP 3: Set the foundation in place by layering a sheer yellow-toned powder on top of it with a cotton ball. Wipe off the excess yellow powder—which helps blend the foundation into the skin tone—with a brush.

IT DOESN'T MATTER WHAT TYPE YOU WERE BORN WITH,

TREAT YOUR SKIN RIGHT!

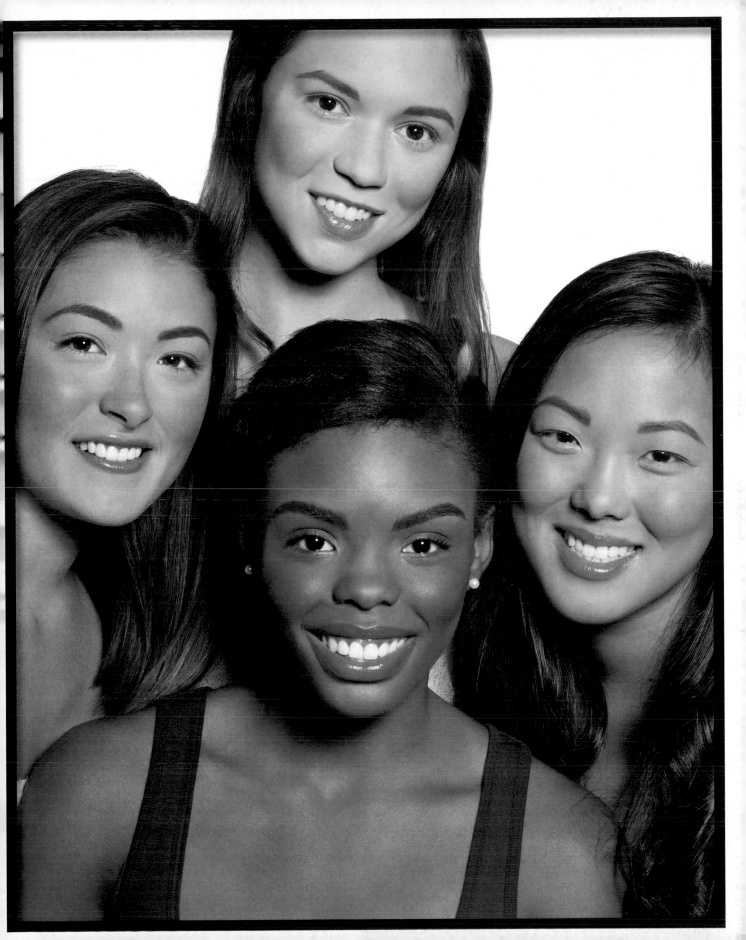

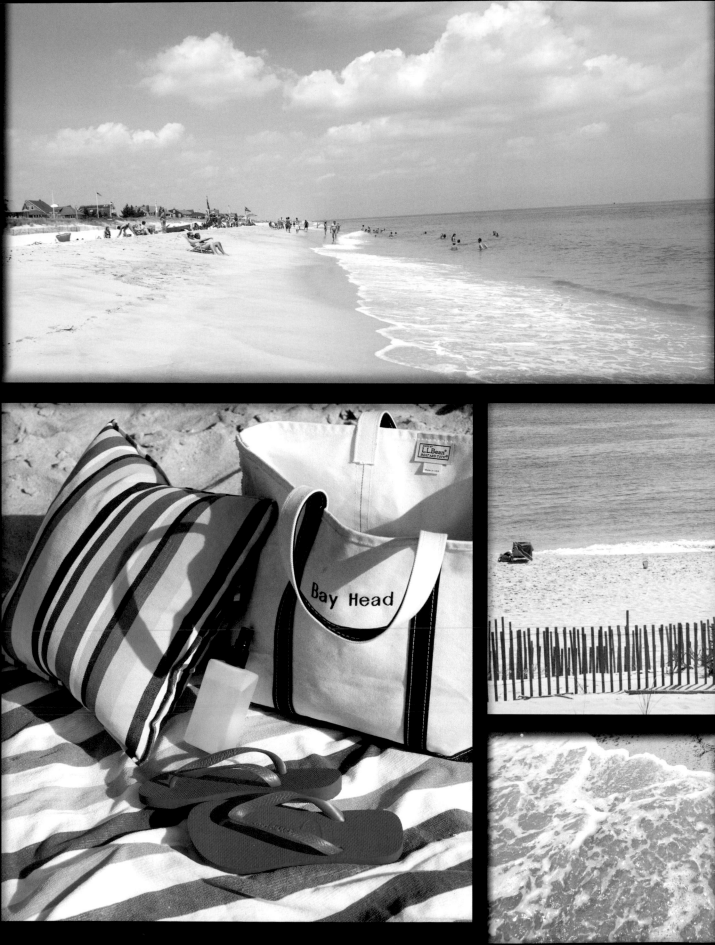

sun blast

File this under the "What-Not-to-Do" section: once, when I was a teen, I took an empty cardboard box, lined it with silver foil, put baby oil and iodine all over my body, and laid out in it under the sun! That's how intense I was about getting tan. If that sounds insane, well, it was. We didn't know how bad the sun was for your skin (or that smoking was bad for you either).

Overexposure to the sun's harmful UVA and UVB rays can cause not only premature wrinkles but also skin cancer later on in life. Regardless, lots of people are still into tanning. Look, I get it. Think about when you put shorts on that first day of summer—scary. A little bit of sun hides a lot of imperfections and gives a healthy glow. The key is to protect yourself because the damage you prevent as a teen will do more for your skin than any wrinkle cream later on.

THE SCIENCE OF SPF

SPF, which stands for *sun protection factor*, is seriously confusing. The sunscreen aisle at the drugstore or chemist has more numbers than math class. SPF tells you how much protection you are getting against UVB rays—those are the ones that cause burns and skin cancer. The number on the bottle tells you how much longer you can stay in the sun after using the sunscreen. Let's say you normally burn after being in the sun for 20 minutes. If you wear an SPF of 10, then you multiply the SPF (10) by how long you can normally stay in the sun (20 minutes) to come up with 200 minutes (the new amount of time it'll take until you burn). That's in a perfect world, and we all know there's no such thing.

The fairer you are, the higher the SPF number you'll need. A bottle of sunscreen with SPF 60 is not double 30, not even close. Most people should wear SPF 15 on the face during the colder months. In the summer months, on the beach or outside playing sports, you should wear at least SPF 30.

APPLY RIGHT

SPF doesn't mean anything if you don't do a good job of applying it. You need a teaspoon of sunscreen for your face and about three tablespoons for your body. Try measuring that out to get an idea of the amount. It'll seem like a lot at first.

Apply it 20 minutes before you go in the sun. The exception is any protection with titanium or zinc—those block light from your skin. Every product needs to be reapplied every two hours, or more if you are swimming or sweating.

Sunscreen isn't just for your nose and shoulders. Make sure it gets into the hairline and all around the ears (there's a lot of skin cancer there because people never think to put SPF on them). The tops of the feet really hurt if burned. And don't forget the lips. There are loads of great lip balms with SPF protection in all sorts of shades.

fake it, don't bake it

Love that sun-kissed look? So do I. Luckily, you don't have to damage your skin to get it. Bronzers and self-tanners can give you the same great glow. Here's how to keep it real when it comes to a fake tan.

BRONZER

Powder is my favorite formula for bronzer because it's pretty much mistake proof and goes on quickly. Take a short, flat, fluffy brush and dust the powder bronzer wherever you typically get sun—the forehead, cheeks, nose, chin, neck, and chest. The trick is to make sure it's blended on the side. You can layer the application to get more color. Bronzers in cream formulas give a dewy look, while gels are very sheer and better for oily skin. Use your fingers to apply these formulas in the same way you would powder.

When it comes to choosing the shade, the most natural-looking bronzers have brown tones with some red. Stay away from anything that's orange or frosted, or you will get that dreaded fake-tan look. Most products come in a range of shades from light to dark. Follow the way your skin tans in real life. So if you turn a dark brown in the sun, go with the dark shade. Don't mess with your natural skin tone or you will just wind up looking orange.

SELF-TANNER

These two little words conjure up scary images of Day-Glo skin. But it doesn't have to be this way. Self-tanner can provide pretty color that lasts for a few days. It's important to start with smooth skin, so make sure to exfoliate all over before hitting the bottle. Test a little bit of the product on the inside of your arm to check for any allergic reactions before putting it anywhere near your face. The secret to successful self-tanning is starting with a very thin layer. Wait until the color sets and you've checked it out to see if you want to do another layer. Don't forget your ears and neck, but be careful to steer clear of your eyes. Once you're done, wash your hands well. Make sure you wait until the self-tanner is completely absorbed before you get dressed. If you find any streaks or the shade is too dark, rub a gentle exfoliant over the darker patches and then moisturize the area of skin to remedy the problem.

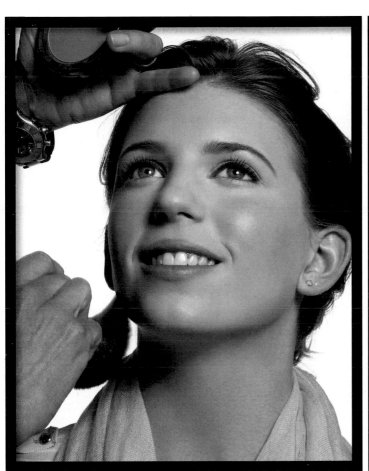

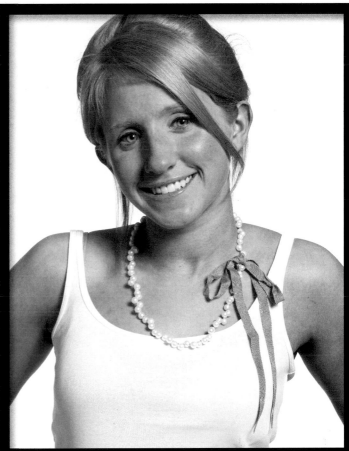

Because Katie has a porcelain complexion, she needs a glow that isn't bronzy. A typical bronzer would appear too dark or orange on her skin. Instead, a bronzer in pinkish and peachy tones that's highlighted with gold flecks gives her skin a completely natural flush.

Aviva also has porcelain skin (I love beautiful pale skin). But she has decided to use a self-tanner because a little color gives her confidence. It's important that the self-tanner looks natural and not too orange. The secret to her sun-kissed glow is to add a little bit of soft bronzer on the cheeks.

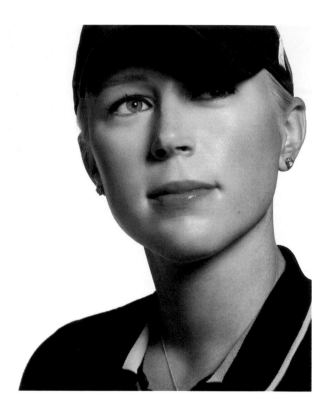

porcelain beauties

You know who you are. You get burned if someone even mentions the word "sun." No matter how light the bronzer or self-tanner is, it just makes you look weird. But, you can still get a pretty glow. Skip self-tanners and opt for a soft pink or apricot blush to warm up your complexion. For a special glow, choose a blush with flecks of gold. On your body, always wear a high SPF when you go outside.

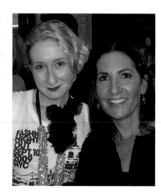

My favorite porcelain beauty, *Vogue* editor Sarah Brown. Only pinks for her.

shop like a pro

There's a sunscreen out there for everyone. There are powders, foundations, moisturizers, lip balms, and lotions, all with SPF. I'm big into protecting my skin because I'm in the sun all the time—whether watering my garden or watching my son's twelve-hour lacrosse tournaments.

When I'm running around in the city, I apply a high-end moisturizer with SPF. I'm usually in a crazy rush, so I use a moisturizer with SPF that I make, which is also tinted. That way I get protection, moisturizer, and foundation—all in one. When I'm playing golf or doing any kind of outdoor activity, I trust heavy-duty sunscreens from Bullfrog or Coppertone and always wear a baseball hat.

HAIR AWAY

Getting rid of unwanted hair is a lifelong battle. Luckily, there are a lot of weapons you can add to your arsenal.

Shaving is one of the simplest, cheapest, and least painful methods of temporary hair removal. It also requires the most maintenance—often daily shaving. For the closest shave, soften hair before you start by using soap rather than shaving cream (a dollop of hair conditioner works great in a pinch). Replace blades frequently, and shave at the end of your shower, when your pores are opened up.

Waxing lasts longer than shaving but costs a lot more when you get it done professionally. You save money with at-home waxing kits, but you'll need to be tough when it comes to ripping the wax off your own body with strips of cloth or paper. Warning: ingrown hairs are common when you wax your bikini line (they can also occur when you shave that sensitive area). Don't pick at the red bumps; this will only make them worse. Treat ingrowns by exfoliating the area with a sudsy loofah or using a product called Tend Skin after you get out of the shower. If the problem is really bad, a doctor can prescribe a topical cortisone gel.

Tweezing is great for grooming eyebrows or getting rid of stray hairs that pop up every now and again on your face. Wide-grip slanted tweezers are the easiest to use. Reduce the pain of plucking by doing it right after you get out of the shower. Pluck the hair as close as you can to the root and pluck it in the direction of the growth so you don't just break off the hair at the surface.

Electrolysis permanently gets rid of hair by sending electricity to the hair follicle, basically killing it. This method is pretty pricey and also painful—a metal needle is inserted into the skin. It also takes a long time because each follicle needs to be zapped.

Laser hair removal is similar to electrolysis, but instead of electricity, it uses an invisible beam of light to penetrate and destroy the hair follicle. The laser beam finds the follicle by first identifying the melanin, or the dark color of the hair. That's why light-skinned people with dark hair have the best results. Laser hair removal isn't great for people with dark skin or those with light skin and light hair since the laser will not be able to target the follicle. It doesn't hurt, but like electrolysis, it's an expensive option.

INTERVIEW: DR. JOELY KAUFMAN
DOCTOR'S ORDERS

Dr. Joely Kaufman—a renowned dermatologist and director of laser at the University of Miami Miller School of Medicine—has seen a lot of different kinds of skin problems and solutions. Here's what she wants every teen to know.

How do you know when your acne is bad enough to see a dermatologist?

Start with over-the-counter medications. Before you invest in an expensive solution, read the ingredients in the products. Some expensive medications have the same exact ingredients in the same percentages as the cheaper ones. If those medicines don't work, then you should visit a doctor.

What are some cool treatments doctors have for acne?

In-office glycolic or salicylic acid peels are helpful in controlling acne, but they don't replace traditional therapies. There are also new light and laser treatments for acne, which treat the bacteria on the skin. The advantage of peels and some of the lasers is that they can also improve the dark marks and scars left by acne. These treatments are not covered by most medical insurances, making them somewhat costly at times. The lasers and light devices tend to be more expensive than peels.

What are some other common skin problems you see in teens?

I see a lot of melasma—brown spots usually over the cheekbones, forehead, or upper lip—that is caused by hormones and sun exposure. To treat it, there are skin lighteners like glycolic acid, but sunblock is the first step. Some girls come in with tiny bumps on the backs of their thighs or arms called keratosis pilaris. It's a hereditary condition that comes from plugging of the hair follicle. To minimize the look of the bumps, try using a loofah in the shower and an exfoliating moisturizer that has lactic acid or urea.

What does smoking do to your skin?

It breaks down collagen. We know that people who smoke heal less quickly than those who don't smoke because they have reduced blood flow. The lines around the mouth also become more pronounced.

What do you think about tanning beds?

They are horrible not only because you are sitting under the worst rays that the sun has to offer but you are also sitting on a piece of equipment that lots of people have used. You have no idea how clean it is. You also don't know the dose you are getting. You can come out a raisin.

What are the consequences of not using sun protection?

Skin cancer rates are increasing. It is a serious problem, not to be taken lightly. It's curable in many cases, but when they have to cut out half your cheek to get rid of the cancer, you are also talking about a real cosmetic issue.

Are hats good for keeping the rays off your skin?

A hat is not a substitute for sun protection. Baseball hats offer sun protection for the forehead, but they aren't so great for the sides of the face and the nose when you are looking up. Tightly woven wide-brimmed hats are better, but I don't see many teenagers wearing those.

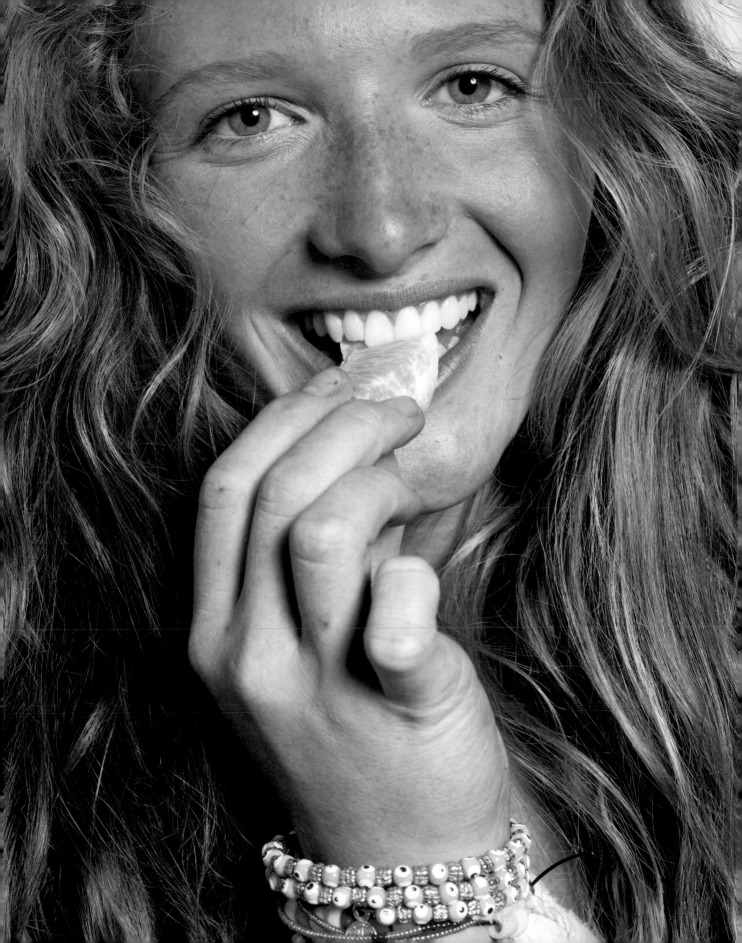

4

BEAUTY FROM THE INSIDE OUT

One of my favorite sayings is that happiness is the best cosmetic for beauty. And one of the best ways I know to be happy is to take great care of yourself by exercising, eating right, sleeping enough, and drinking plenty of water. Honestly, the healthier you are, the better and prettier you'll look and feel.

I practice what I preach. On days when I've taken a spinning class, polished off a CamelBak of cold water, and fueled up on a big salad topped by fresh fish, I'm unstoppable. But I wasn't always such a fitness and nutritional nut. When I was a teen, I thought sugar was one of the major food groups, and the only way you would catch me running was if it was away from gym class. It took me a long time to change my habits, but I'm so glad I did because I've never felt better. So even if you are a fast-food fanatic or have never stepped on a treadmill, there's a way to start.

Taking care of your body increases your energy and brainpower so that tasks like homework are easier to perform. A healthy lifestyle will show on the outside but the most amazing product of your new beauty regimen is how incredible you will feel on the inside.

food, glorious food

I have watched my weight my whole life. When I was a teen, I didn't accept my body type. I wanted to be taller, skinnier, someone else. So I tried to change with a bunch of fad diets. I tortured myself drinking stuff such as apple cider vinegar and cod-liver oil. Save yourself time, money, suffering, and pounds. Yes, pounds. Fad diets not only don't work but they can add more weight after you come off them. It took me a while to get it, but all you need to do is eat simple, wholesome foods and give up trying to look like you stepped out of a magazine. It has been a positive thing for me to eat healthy. Food really affects mood. The better you eat, the easier it is to deal with everything from homework to emotions to parents. So, love food and love yourself.

for the total beginner

I don't expect anyone to change overnight. It's really about learning better eating habits and making small steps. If you are just starting out, try one of these suggestions. See how it makes you feel, and hopefully you'll be inspired to make more changes.

AVOID FRIED FOODS. There are so many kinds of food out there; you won't go hungry if you avoid those that are fried.

BRING LUNCH TO SCHOOL. When you make food yourself, it is mostly always more nutritious than if you buy it. Brown-bagging it takes a little more effort, but it will pay off in the long run.

REPLACE THE MAYONNAISE. On your favorite sandwich, use a really good French mustard, and try a great crisp green apple for dessert. You won't sacrifice in flavor what you give up in fat.

SKIP THE SODA. Replace all those empty calories with thirst-quenching water. If you crave the carbonation, try a flavored sparkling water.

meal plan

It's taken years of experience for me to learn the right eating choices. If I look at a piece of cake or a rich cookie, I still want to eat it. I know, though, I won't feel good after I do. So I'll skip it. The more you eat healthy foods, the more you'll crave them (although when I walk into my Aunt Alice's house, there's nothing that will keep me from eating one, or three, of her famous toffee squares). When it comes to the topic of nutrition, you can quickly drive yourself crazy with information about food that's constantly changing in magazines or on TV. But if you follow a few core principles, you'll be eating right in no time.

EAT TONS OF VEGGIES AND LOTS OF FRUIT: This food group should actually be the bulk of your diet. At any meal, look at your plate and see what's taking up the most room. Is it a big green salad with chicken on top? (Great!) Or is it a burger and fries with nothing green in sight? (Not so great.) Aim for a lot of color—yellow corn, red peppers, green broccoli, blueberries. You get the idea.

EAT WHOLE GRAINS: This essential food group not only gives you a lot of energy but is low in fat and delivers many important nutrients. It also tastes way better than the white stuff once you switch over. Whole grain means that both the inside and outer covering of the grain—such as wheat—is part of the food. Processed flours don't have the outer covering, which makes food like white bread a lot lighter, and a lot less nutritious. Try to eat whole-grain versions of bread, pasta, and cereal whenever you can. If you want to get adventurous, branch out and try less-common grains like wild rice, buckwheat, bulgur, or barley (I love quinoa).

EAT LEAN PROTEIN: Opt for chicken, fish, or pork. Beans, nuts, and tofu are also great ways to get proteins, which are part of every cell in our bodies. The protein in our body is constantly being broken down and needs to be replaced by protein we eat. Eggs, cheese, and red meat, which are higher in saturated fat, are fine in moderation.

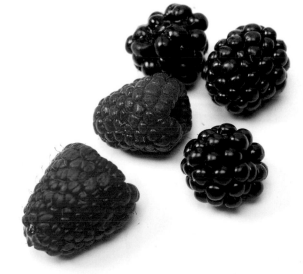

shop like a pro

Junk food is more than just candy bars and fast-food burgers. Some foods, like certain cereals, bread, or even nutrition bars, seem like they are good for you. But actually they are filled with processed ingredients, chemicals, and hidden calories. I don't care what the package looks like or what the ad says; the only way to know what you are eating is to read the ingredients on the label.

AVOID FOODS THAT HAVE A VERY LONG LIST OF INGREDIENTS WITH NAMES YOU DON'T RECOGNIZE OR CAN'T PRONOUNCE. When my kids wanted cookies and the really nutritious stuff wouldn't do, I bought them Walkers from England because they have only three ingredients: sugar, wheat, and butter. Those aren't exactly health food, and they do have sugar, but I also know what the ingredients are. Foods with more than five ingredients (especially if you have no idea what they are) are most likely highly processed and filled with chemicals.

STAY AWAY FROM HIGH-FRUCTOSE CORN SYRUP. This is hard because the sweetener is found in everything from soda to bread to ketchup. It is so common because it extends the shelf life of processed foods and is inexpensive. The problem is that most processed foods made with high-fructose corn syrup are high in calories and low in nutritional value.

ENRICHED FLOUR IS NOT A WHOLE GRAIN. When flour is enriched, it has been processed, and some nutrients and vitamins are added later. It's much better to eat foods with whole grains (look for the word *whole* on the package, and make sure it appears early in the ingredient list).

treat yourself

It's fine to eat what you love, even if it's not terrific for you, as long as you keep it to a low percentage. When it comes to eating, I now eat 90 percent good and 10 percent not so good. It wasn't always this way. As a kid, my junk-food percentage was way higher.

You have to eat what you love or else you will feel deprived and want those things even more. Plus, fries, cake, and cookies are all delicious. My food of choice is definitely pizza. But I order the thinner, crispier kind with veggies, and I don't do it every day.

When I indulge, I make sure it counts. I love french fries, but they have to be really, really good. If it's some fat, overcooked potato, forget it. When I travel to Paris for work, I will eat delicious buttery croissants and Brie cheese. When you are treating yourself, go for high quality and enjoy. The message is: Think before you eat, go slowly, and stop a bit before you're full (it really takes twenty minutes for the body to register feelings of satiety).

BAD

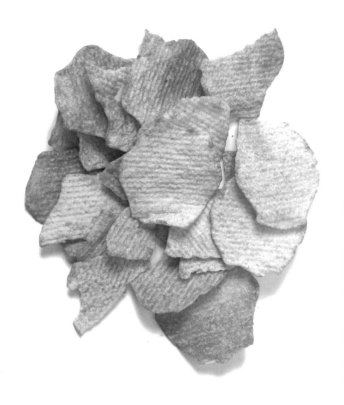

BAD

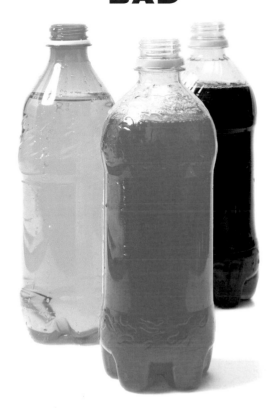

GOOD

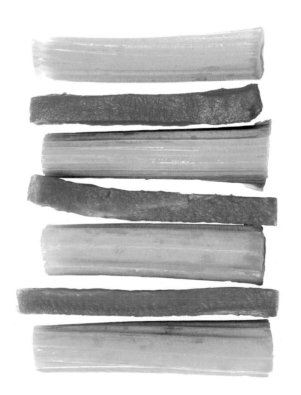

GOOD

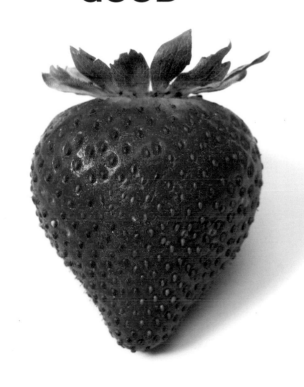

WHAT'S ON BOBBI'S PLATE

Check out how much my diet has changed by comparing a typical day of eating for me when I was a teen and one now. If I can do it, so can you.

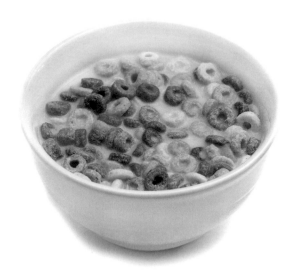

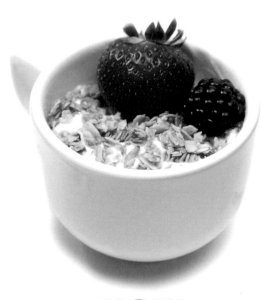

THEN

BREAKFAST
A bowl of some sugary cereal with milk

LUNCH
Grilled-cheese sandwich and cream-of-tomato soup

DINNER
Canned peas, a hamburger, and some kind of oven-baked potatoes

DESSERT
Cake, cookies, or ice cream

NOW

BREAKFAST
A protein shake, a small cup of oatmeal with berries, or a poached egg and whole-grain toast

LUNCH
Chopped salad with tons of veggies and some kind of protein in it and brown rice crackers

DINNER
A piece of fish, broccoli, and whole-wheat pasta

DESSERT
A very small vanilla frozen yogurt with blueberries or dark chocolate chips

water works

Drinking water is essential to being healthy. We are made up of mostly water (on average, 60 percent of your body weight is water). It also brings important nutrients into our cells and flushes bad toxins out. Yes, those are the vital stats. But from a beauty expert's perspective, staying hydrated simply makes skin look great. It gives your face a dewy, glowing appearance, and your eyes will be clearer. Plus, when you down a lot of H_2O, you have more energy and your brain works better.

FOR THE TOTAL BEGINNER

If you aren't big into water, try what I do when I'm not in the mood to drink plain water. I add a splash of cranberry juice (without sugar), a touch of lemon, or even a hint of lemonade. A bit of flavor makes water go down easier. In my studio, we always have a big glass pitcher filled with water flavored by cucumber slices. It is so delicious and refreshing.

DRINK PLAN

HOW MUCH YOU SHOULD DRINK: You need to replenish the water you lose naturally through normal body functions such as breathing, sweating, and going to the bathroom. While everyone's body is a little different, a good goal is to drink eight 8-ounce glasses of water a day. You lose even more water when you exercise or it's really hot out. Another good rule to follow is to drink enough so that you never get thirsty. By the time you feel thirsty, you are already mildly dehydrated.

DRINK UP: It can be hard to remember to drink enough water. I like to carry a bottle around with me so that hydration is never far away. A good policy is to drink at least a glass before you exercise and one after. I also like to drink a glass before I eat. Sometimes when you think you are hungry, you are actually thirsty. When it's cold, you will always find me with a reusable Thermos filled with peppermint or chamomile tea. As long as the tea is herbal, it counts.

THE GREAT BOTTLE DEBATE: There's a time and a place for bottled water. But bottled water is really bad for the environment. Not only does it take energy and resources to make plastic bottles, a lot of them also wind up in landfills. Go green by getting a reusable drinking bottle that you can refill with cooler or filtered tap water. My favorite kind is made by CamelBak because it has a built-in straw—which a nutritionist told me allows you drink more water faster. There are also aluminum reusable bottles in all kinds of great colors that keep water cool during your day.

move it

I was the kid who always got notes to get out of gym class. Field hockey was big back then. Hated it. I didn't like swimming, running, or anything that made me sweat. It wasn't until I got to college—when I wanted to lose weight without starving myself—that I really started exercising. What I found was similar to eating right. The more I worked out, the more I loved and needed it. Now sports are my passion. I exercise to be healthy and for fun. Whether it's running or doing downward dog in yoga, moving makes me feel good, reduces stress, opens up my mind, and allows me to be more creative.

FOR THE TOTAL BEGINNER

Are you the person who is always picked last for any team? Don't be embarrassed—I was too. That doesn't mean you can't get your blood pumping. Exercising can be a simple, equipment-free experience. Resolve to walk at a pace that gets your heart rate up for fifteen minutes, three times a week. After a couple of weeks, add five minutes on to your walk. Keep it up and see how far you go.

EXERCISE PLAN

PUT IT ON YOUR CALENDAR: This is pretty basic, but you have to make time for exercise. Include it as part of your regular schedule, just like doing homework or making plans with friends. Even on days when you don't have time to go to the gym or take a class, sneak in a little physical activity. Walk up the stairs instead of taking an elevator or have your parents drop you off a little farther. It all adds up.

FIND YOUR STYLE: There are so many different ways to exercise. Open up the gym doors and free your inner athlete. For me a typical week includes spinning, weight training, running, walking, and yoga. But there are so many other activities like skateboarding, jumping rope, dancing, or hiking. Do what inspires you and you'll have a better chance of sticking to it.

HAVE FUN: Even if you've found a sport you are passionate about be open to trying new things. Changing your exercise routine keeps you from becoming bored. It also keeps your body from hitting a plateau by using different muscle groups. Great music will liven up any workout. Make playlists with songs that will get you pumped. Some people are inspired by cute workout clothes. One of my favorite things to do is work out with a friend or my family. I can't always chat (especially if I'm out of breath), but it's nice to be active together.

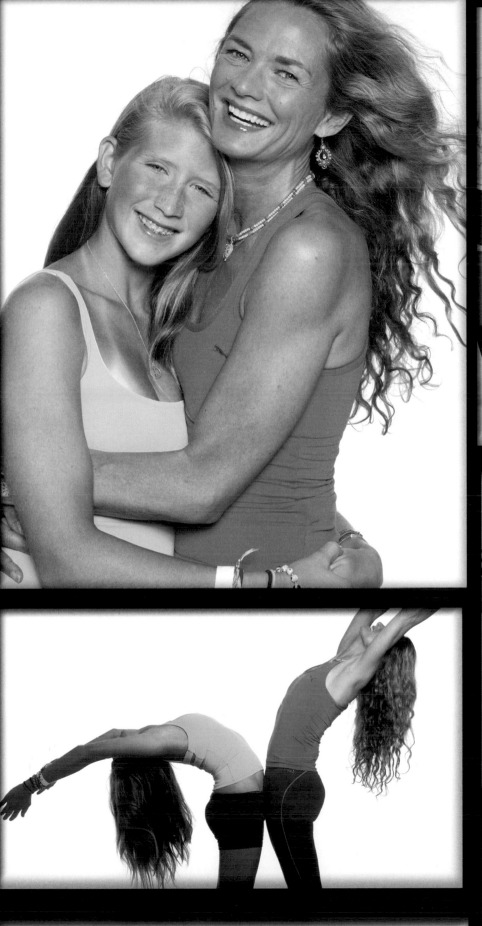
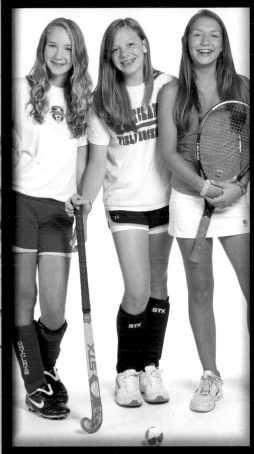
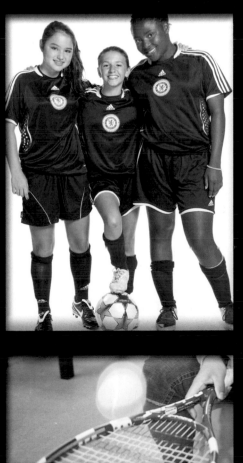

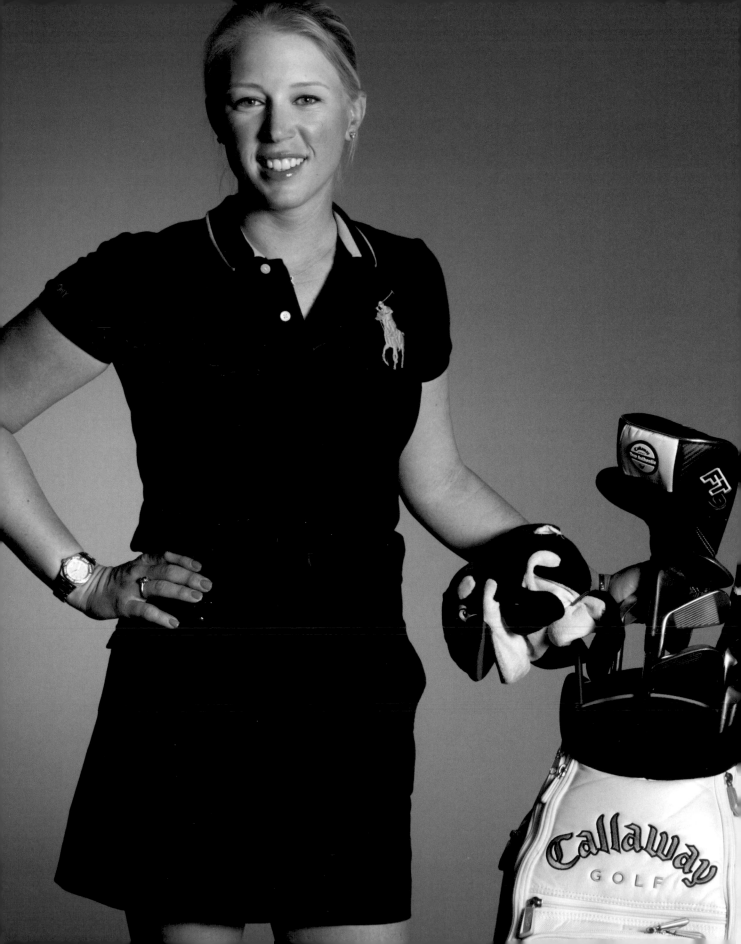

INTERVIEW: MORGAN PRESSEL
GOLF'S GOLDEN GIRL

The youngest-ever winner of an LPGA major tournament, Morgan has worked hard to reach number four in the Women's World Golf Rankings. Her biggest beauty challenge is keeping her skin from frying during an average of eight hours a day in the hot sun!

When did you know you wanted to be a pro golfer?

In 2001, when I was twelve, I was the youngest person to qualify for the U.S. Women's Open. I just went for the experience, and lo and behold, I won the qualifier. When I played in the Open, I realized that is what I wanted to do. I was playing against the people I grew up idolizing. I had only been playing for four years. To think the crowd was watching me play was pretty special.

What's a typical day in your life like?

I spend thirty weeks a year on the road, on the low end, playing about twenty-three tournaments. The rest of the time, I'm either doing functions or charity events. When I'm on the road, it's busy. Practicing and playing golf takes up most of my day. Then I might want to work out a little bit, have a nice meal with family and friends, and then go to bed.

How much do you play golf?

Nine holes takes two and a half hours; eighteen holes takes about five hours. I usually practice a couple hours before as well. So I'm playing between a six- and nine-hour day on the road.

And then you *also* work out?

If I can find time to get to the gym three or four times a week on the road, I'm pretty happy. I do light weights for toning and lots of cardio. I love to spin when I'm home, but it's hard to find a spinning class on the road. Some golfers work out before and after their rounds every day. That just amazes me.

Are you an exercise freak?

I don't love exercising. I have to motivate myself to do that. You just do it. There is no substitute. Sitting on your butt will not make the muscles stronger. You are not burning calories on the couch watching TV.

Is golf a good workout?

More than anything golf takes mental endurance. You have to be in good shape to play on hilly courses and in heat. But more than the physical stuff, honing your golf skills is a serious mental task. It is such a mental game. You have to be able to hold your focus for five hours, not get down on yourself when you are playing poorly, come back from bad shots, and so many other things.

What's your diet like?

I'm eating chips and dip right now [laughs]. Travel days are my fat days. I'm more lenient with myself. I have three weaknesses: french fries, chocolate, and Coke. Terrible, terrible, and terrible. I have an idea of what I should and shouldn't be eating. I try to have a mix that includes enough protein, natural sugar, vegetables, and wheat.

Do you eat any differently before a tournament?

I just make sure I have eggs in the morning for extra protein.

How do you deal with the attention that comes with fame?

Luckily, we don't have paparazzi in golf. I'm a normal person who just happens to have a little bit of media attention. Some people hate it. For me, the problem is when no one wants to talk to me. I would rather have someone ask me for an autograph. There will come a day when no one wants your autograph. And that will be a sad one.

What's your style like?

I'm preppy more than anything. I'm a Palm Beacher. Pinks and greens and all that fun stuff. I wear a polo shirt and pop my collar. I'm *that* dork.

What's your beauty regimen?

I wear tons of sunscreen. I didn't used to, so I'm nervous about the future of my skin. There were the days when I would forget it or leave it off on purpose to even out my tan. I spend nine hours in the sun! Growing up and taking care of your body is all part of the process. When you are young, you think you are invincible. I felt that way. I was that person who was too cool to wear sunscreen. Those days are gone.

What kind of sunscreen do you use?

I've tried every sunscreen on the planet. I use Neutrogena Active Sport in SPF 70. It is not oily and sticky and doesn't come off when you sweat.

What's the best thing about being a pro golfer?

Being different. I play a game for a living. There aren't many people who get to travel all over the world and have lots and lots of contacts all over the globe. I get to meet cool people like Bobbi. It's a challenge every day.

"EXPERIENCE IS THE BEST WAY TO WORK ON YOUR MENTAL SKILLS"

–MORGAN PRESSEL

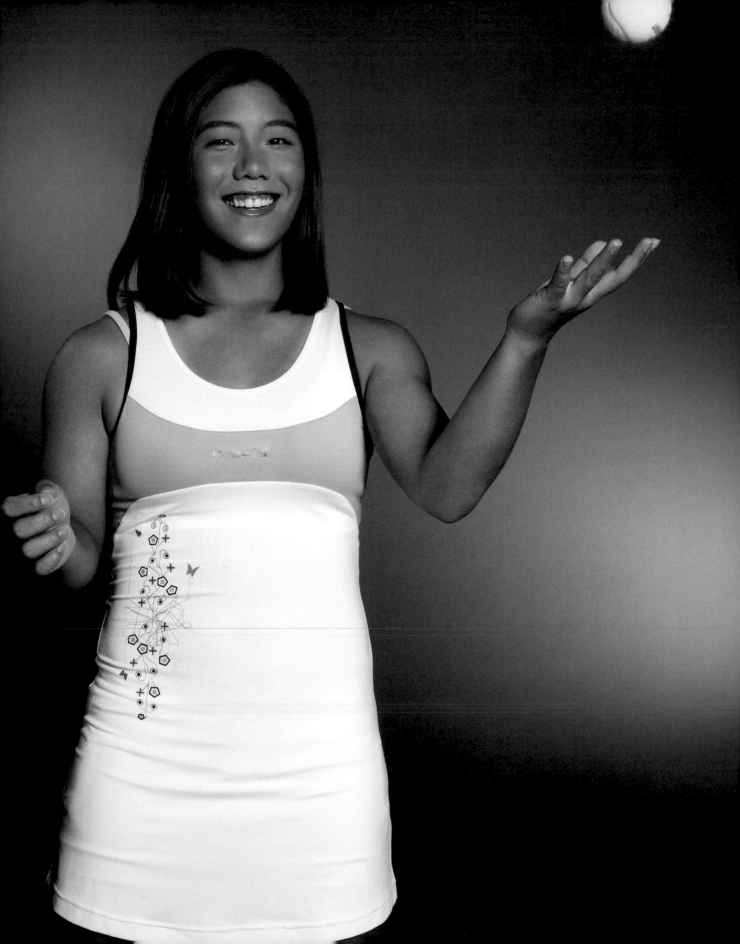

INTERVIEW: KRISTIE AHN
THE TENNIS STAR WHO'S ALWAYS GAME

This Jersey girl transitioned from a soccer player to a tennis player around eight years old, which is kind of a late start. But Kristie quickly made up for lost time, consistently placing at national events ever since she turned twelve. She broke out of the pack in 2008, winning her first pro match at the age of fifteen. With school in the morning and tennis all afternoon, that doesn't leave much time for shopping. But that doesn't bother Kristie.

How much do you practice tennis?

In the summer, I practice four hours a day, five days a week. Another big part of my summer is devoted to general fitness. I will also play soccer or run around a track for a workout. In the winter, I play tennis an hour and a half every day.

How do you fuel up for all that exercise?

Carbs are good. I try to eat whole grains. Pasta is one of my favorite things to eat. Sometimes I want junk food. But I know if I eat it before I play, I won't do as well. In the summer I find myself eating a lot. It's not bad though because I spend a lot of time playing and working out. . . . At my old high school, some of the girls would eat tiny amounts. I found it disturbing.

Do you worry about your appearance, especially since you are now in the public eye?

I don't wear makeup or do my hair. I don't like to. Sports is not about how you look. It's about how good you play and your sportsmanship. I would be the guys' favorite girl in gym because I tried hard. Guys will like you a lot more when you play sports.

How would you describe your style?

I wear sweatshirts and sweatpants all day. Jeans are for nice occasions. My mom always tries to take me shopping, I want to relax when I get a break from tennis. My mom's like, "Why can't you be more like a typical girl?" I tell her I'm saving her money by not buying clothes. Everyone is different.

What do you think is one of your most attractive qualities?

I like to think of myself as someone who makes people laugh. Even when I lost at the U.S. Open, I tried to get the crowd behind me.

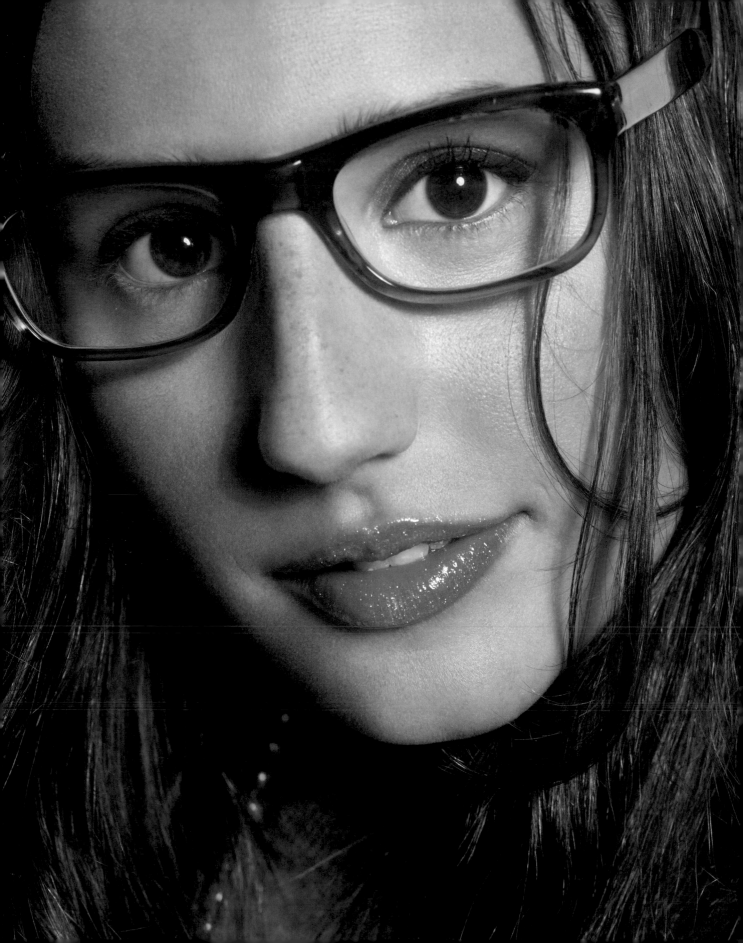

5

BE WHO YOU ARE

Everyone wants to be pretty. But to be amazing and special is about so much more than just your looks. It takes style, substance, kindness, and confidence. It takes understanding and then loving who you are. The world is a melting pot. Everybody's got a story— becoming comfortable with your own is the challenge. It's something you need to learn. Whether you are tall, small, a celebrity, or a sister, I want you to celebrate the qualities that make you unique. They are what inspire me. They should inspire you, too.

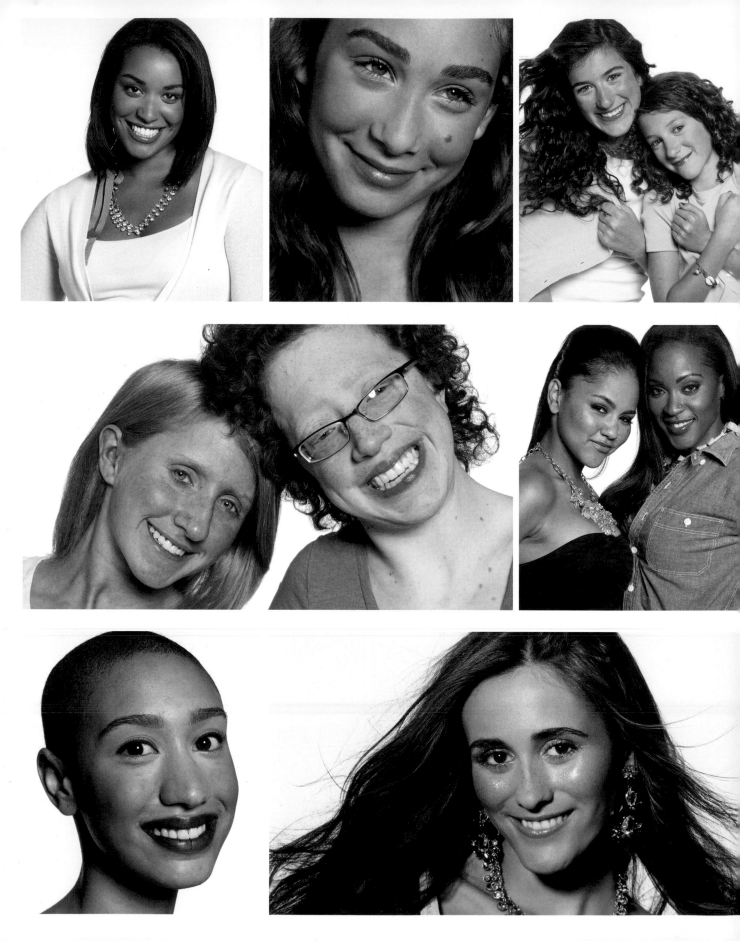

be tall

When Lauren was a kid, she didn't like being tall. Really tall. "In the playground, I could grab the monkey bars without even stretching," says Lauren, who reconsidered her feelings on her height after getting into sports around the fourth grade. "After I realized I could use my height to my advantage, I began to appreciate it more," she says. Lauren definitely took full advantage of her 5 feet 11 inches: the high school senior is headed to college to play basketball.

Sports helped Lauren feel better about her body type, and so did *America's Next Top Model,* which she says "made being tall cool." But sometimes she's still not totally confident. "Because I'm an athlete, I'm bigger than most girls. Sometimes I get insecure in a bathing suit," she admits. "I feel big."

To keep walking tall, she surrounds herself with people who don't judge her. That includes her boyfriend, who is an inch shorter than Lauren. "I feel so comfortable with my boyfriend that height is not an issue," she says. It did become an issue, however, when prom rolled around. After a lot of shoe shopping, Lauren settled on a pair of strappy, black patent leather Prada shoes with a thick four-inch heel that would put her five inches above her guy. "My boyfriend said, 'Don't wear them,'" Lauren remembers. "But I didn't listen to him. I thought, 'I'll look so hot.' I'm such a diva." In the end, Lauren took off her heels within the first ten minutes of prom. "Not because of my boyfriend," she laughs. "But because they were so uncomfortable."

be small

That's me. Small. Petite. However you want to put it. I have struggled my whole life to accept that I'm only 5 feet tall. I feel so much bigger. Maybe it's my outsize personality (or maybe it's just the platforms I wear whenever possible). All I know is that certain beauty role models I have make being a shorty much easier to take. I've been a longtime fan of Natalie Portman, who wears her small stature with such grace that it's astonishing. But Natalie's super-slim, and I'm not. Scarlett Johansson is a great model for me. At 5 feet 2 inches, she's got a couple inches over me, however, we share the same womanly curves. Scarlett owns her body and celebrates her shape with flattering pencil skirts and old-Hollywood bodices. The fashion world has also found a new love of breasts and hips with Scarlett: she's landed some of the biggest fashion ad campaigns around. There's a positive beauty role model out there for every size of woman. Find a star, athlete, or singer with your body type whom you admire when you need some personal encouragement.

be a good sister

Aviva can be pretty critical about her own looks: she'll complain about her pale skin (although pale is beautiful: think Gwyneth Paltrow). Her younger sister Hannah doesn't see any of that. "She's beautiful. She's my sister," Hannah says. It's a mutual admiration society here. Aviva thinks Hannah has "the most fantastic smile. She really exudes happiness." A big part of Hannah's happiness comes from the support she gets from her sister in everything from encouragement to clothes. "When I'm away, she calls my room the Aviva store," Aviva laughs. "I come home to find her wearing all my clothes." Hannah might crib from Aviva's style, but Aviva's taking a page from her sister's resilience. "She goes to school every day and faces mean kids, who tease her. The fact that she still goes back every day is inspiring," says Aviva, who admires her sister's "willingness to accept people no matter how they treat her. She is always the bigger person."

be a superstar

Shontelle and Kat have a lot in common. They have wanted to be singers ever since they can remember. "You know when babies are born, and they pat them to cry. They patted me and I sang," says Kat, who grew up in the Dominican Republic. Shontelle, who is from Barbados, was inspired by *The Little Mermaid*— "I wanted a voice that was in such demand that the wicked witch would want to steal it."

Both girls have also succeeded in breaking into the really tough business of entertainment. "I'm the dreamer type of girl who thinks there is nothing I can't accomplish," Kat gives as the reason she's made it. "You have to dream big, no matter where you come from."

Now that the singers are stars, Shontelle says, "Life is very different. You have a lot less free time, privacy, and sleep. But a lot more attention." Some of that attention—like having a hit single—is good. And some of it—like vicious rumors on the Internet—is terrible. Criticism "hurts every time," says Shontelle, who will send out a message on Twitter whenever she feels down. "Then my real fans come out to cheer me up. There are a million people who love you for every one who hates you." Or she'll call her mom for a lesson in tough love.

Kat agrees that you need strong people, including your family, around to keep you grounded. She relies on her mom and sisters to tell her when an outfit doesn't look right or someone she thinks is really cool isn't all that. Whatever bumps she encounters, Kat feels blessed for her career. But she gives the most credit to working hard. "I don't know if I believe in luck," she says. "Luck is just preparing yourself for the perfect moment."

be bold

Seta is used to standing out. Her mother's Armenian, and her dad is a mix of African American, Cherokee, and Irish. So no one can ever place her striking and unusual features. "I've gotten Egyptian, Hispanic, Asiatic. I like that people don't know what I am," Seta says. "I like to hear where people think I'm from. They usually think I'm more exotic than I am."

Already a head-turner, Seta started causing whiplash when she shaved off all her hair. "I used to have chin-length hair and straight bangs," she says. "It was time for a change." Hello! Most people would choose to get highlights, not go bald. "I was a little nervous, but with hair I like to be different," Seta explains.

She's not as confident in every area of her life: "I'm a very anxious person. I get insecure about my body sometimes, because I'm a dancer, and being thinner is just easier." Cutting off all her hair (and all the compliments she's received) has made her bolder. "I always wanted to do it, and I finally found the courage."

be you

Grammy Award winner Estelle has always made the most of what she has. Even when she was just a skinny kid growing up in London, she loved fashion but had to settle for "a lot of hand-me-downs from my brother, cousins, and everyone." That didn't stop her from looking great. "I would customize and make it work," she says. "I paid close attention to my auntie's magazines. I was the kid pointing out the most expensive YSL dress, saying, 'When I grow up . . .'"

The R&B singer-songwriter and producer wasn't wrong. She has grown up to wear designer clothes, like Yves Saint Laurent, and hit the top of her profession. Despite how different her life is now, some things have stayed the same since she was a kid, including her obsession with reading and listening to music. "I used to sleep with books under my pillow, which my mum would rotate," she says.

Estelle credits her mom with influencing her on much more than just her reading. "My mum instilled in me that it's not what you look like; it's what your heart is like," she says. "You could be the best-looking girl in school and end up a mess." That philosophy has helped her when the limelight's glow grows harsh. For example, when a blog talks about the lines in her forehead, she focuses on "what have I done to maintain being a nice person versus what Botox I can get."

When she really needs a pick-me-up, Estelle can always turn to her surefire method for feeling beautiful, which is "being in my underwear on a Saturday afternoon, dancing around my house to music I listened to growing up."

be comfortable in your own skin

The first feature Joan notices when she looks at other people is their skin. That's because as someone who suffers from chronic acne, she battles with accepting her own. "You try everything out there—doctors, prescriptions, treatments, over-the-counter products, what people recommend, your own concoctions and formulas," she says. "And at the end of the day, you notice a new zit on your face." After spending so much time, money, and energy, Joan used to find a new break-out completely disheartening. "I use to ask myself over and over, 'Why me? Why do I have such terrible skin? What am I doing wrong?' I would get depressed and not want to go out. I would make myself feel miserable because I didn't like the way my skin looks," Joan explains.

Although she still has acne flare-ups, these days her emotions are under control. Joan has come to realize that no one is scrutinizing her skin the way she is. Sure, she doesn't look her best when she's got pimples, but they are gone in a few days. "It's not permanent," Joan says. When a blemish appears, she copes with it by staying away from the mirror, pretending it's not there, taking a breath, and reminding herself, "It's only temporary." She can also take heart that lots of people, even the world's most beautiful actresses and powerful celebrities, have pimple outbreaks. Just check out the Proactiv commercials with Vanessa Williams, Jessica Simpson, and P. Diddy talking about their bad skin!

Joan also works hard to remind herself, "It doesn't matter how your skin looks. What matters is on the inside. That's what people notice and will remember you for." That's pretty deep. "Beauty lies within," Joan says. "We all age and change, but our personality and attitude are what get us through our lives."

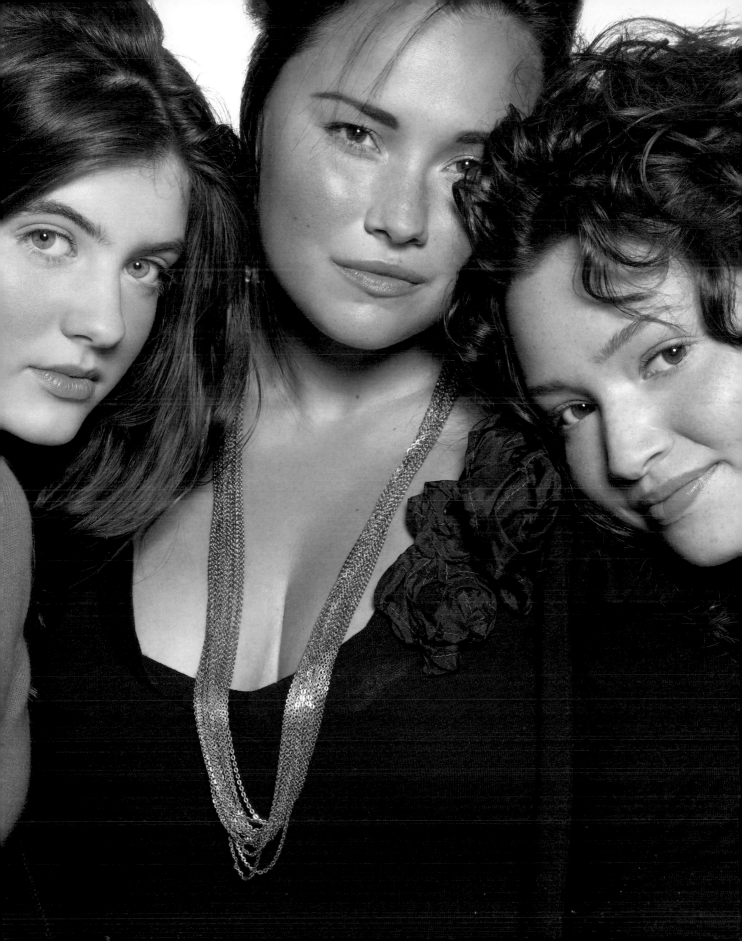

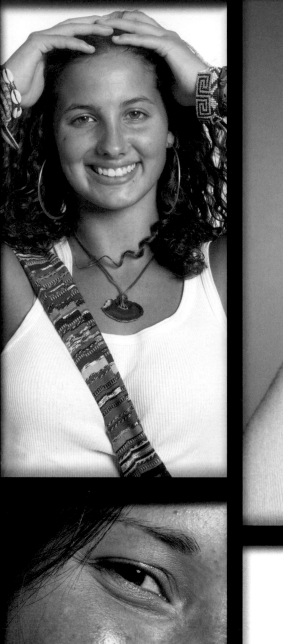
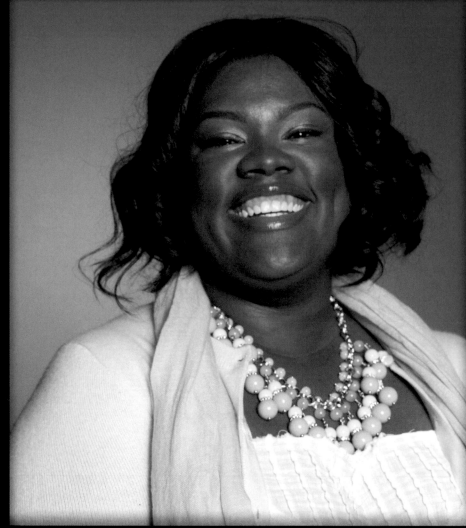
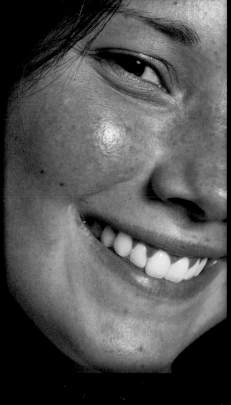
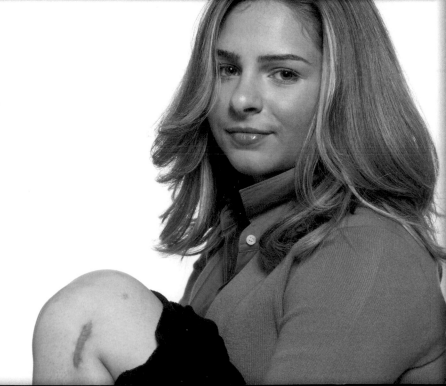

featuring you

Us girls have a love-hate relationship with standing out. We want to stand out from the crowd, have people take notice of us. But often we're embarrassed of our distinguishing features. Things that are extreme and not of the norm—freckles, strong noses, really red hair, really blond hair, really black hair—are where I find beauty.

Every single girl wants to be someone else in some way. I have never met a girl who wouldn't want to trade something about her appearance. Usually, they pick those quirky or interesting features that make them an individual. But when you get older, you see that those traits set you apart, especially if you can work them. Turquoise jewelry dazzles when set against a backdrop of black hair. Ivory skin goes from deathly pale to wonderfully romantic with a swath of pink blush. You get it.

I'm not saying you are going to love every single part of yourself. Everyone's got insecurities. I have seen the most gorgeous girls with the greatest bodies and terrible skin. Or women with amazing eyes and limp hair. But when you find yourself criticizing an aspect of your appearance, take another look. Is it really a liability? Or is it an asset waiting to be discovered?

Don't minimize your unique characteristics. Learn to become comfortable with them by making the most of them. Whether they are features you were born with, like coloring or bone structure, or ones you've acquired for your health, like glasses or braces, or even ones you've chosen, like a piercing, you need to make the best of what you've got. Have fun figuring out what makes you special.

(CLOCKWISE FROM TOP LEFT):

Chloe has a dimple on her cheek that's unique to her; Waltaya's huge smile shows how beyond self-confident she is; Hannah leads an active life— and has a scar on her knee to prove it; Stephanie thinks her pink cheeks are a flaw. I think they are gorgeous.

braces

Rarely do you find a girl who says, "Look at my awesome braces." These are a temporary inconvenience on the road to gorgeousness. The most important element in looking great in your braces is your attitude. You can either wear them with a scowl or a smile (come on, with teeth is fine).

So when you get down about your metal mouth, remember you have braces for a reason. You are lucky your parents got them for you (they are expensive!). Don't forget to wear your rubber bands and your night guard. This is just a moment in time. So you have braces? It's better than crooked teeth.

Okay, now a few beauty pointers when it comes to braces: your lips are probably very dry, so lip gloss and lip balm are way better for you right now than other lip formulas. If you are really freaking out about your braces, or simply don't like them, play up other areas of your face. Get some highlights in your hair or draw attention to your eyes with shimmer and a few extra coats of mascara.

strong noses

I have one and I love them. When I was a kid, my mom thought I should have a nose job, even though I never expressed any kind of insecurity about it. Luckily, I listened to myself and didn't go through with it. I think my nose looks great on my face and wouldn't change a thing about it. There are a number of actresses who have had nose jobs, and frankly, I think they all looked better beforehand. If you really hate your nose, talk to your parents and look into your options. But wait a while before you go through with anything permanent. Once you alter your nose, there is no going back. In the meantime, pick up a copy of *Vogue Italia* and flip through its pages to find stunning women with strong noses for a different perspective and an ego boost.

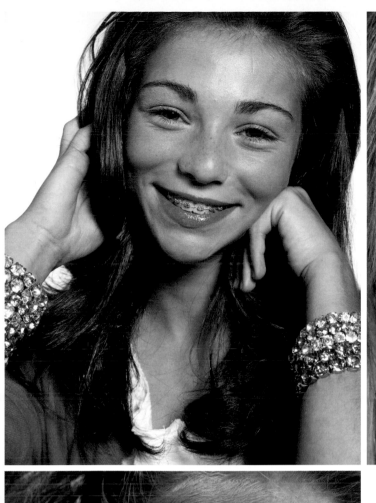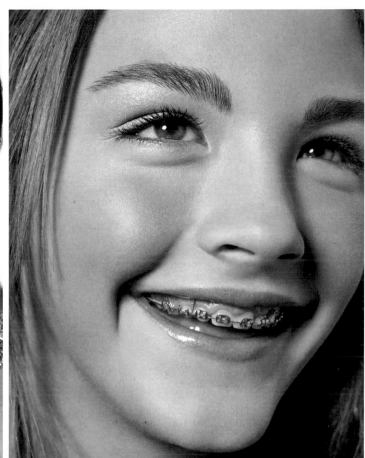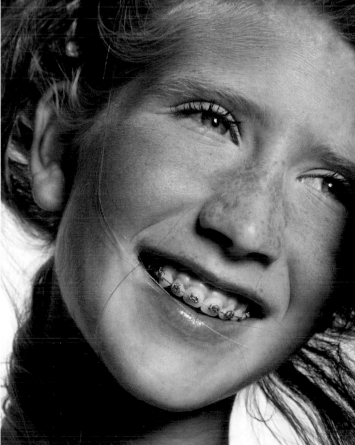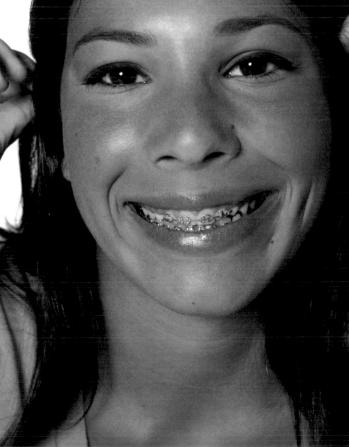

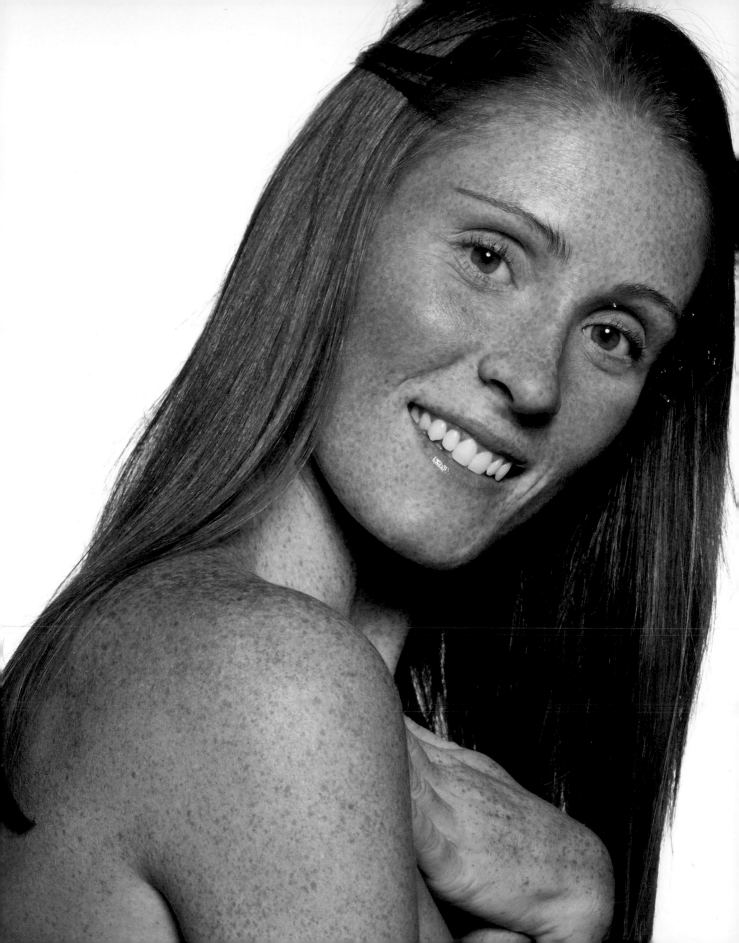

freckles

I love freckles. I can't say it enough. They just look incredible, and they age beautifully. I don't think I've ever met a woman with freckles and wrinkles. Actress Julianne Moore is the ultimate beauty role model when it comes to freckles. Without makeup, she radiates warmth. When she's all glammed up for a premiere, Julianne looks so unique and fabulously gorgeous.

The challenge for girls with Julianne's kind of complexion is finding a foundation that doesn't cover their freckles and make them look pasty. Often, once you put a foundation on, it turns the freckle part ashy and dark. To even out your skin tone, go with a tinted moisturizer in a warm color. If it's between two colors, always go with the darker color. You can also use a sheer foundation everywhere with a cover-up stick for specific spots around the nose.

Often, people with freckles have white or light eyebrows and eyelashes. Softly use makeup to enhance or fill in them in. A freckle-covered redhead with strong mascara, and basically nothing else except a little gloss, is one of the coolest looks around.

glasses

The idea that glasses are for nerds is about as current as wearing a girdle. I wear glasses a lot. Sometimes I hide behind them: if you wake up and you are having a bad beauty day, all you need to do is throw on a big pair of black glasses.

Anyone who wears glasses should look at Tina Fey if they are feeling insecure. She plays with the cliché of the funny smart girl by wearing flattering, chic glasses that come off as cool and pretty.

If you need glasses to see, the best thing to do is have a couple of different styles on hand. I know they are expensive. But if you can swing it, having a strong chunky pair and a more delicate set of frames will afford you more versatility in your outfits and general look.

When it comes to makeup, glasses magnify any product you use. The more definition you do, the more your eyes will stand out. Smudge shadow, liner, and mascara will make your eyes pop out from behind those frames.

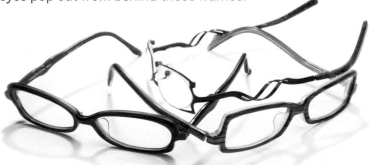

piercings and tattoos

Whatever you do, whether it's a piercing or a tattoo, here is my big warning: It's permanent. It's not going anywhere. What you think is cool when you are fifteen, eighteen, or twenty is going to be with you until you are eighty years old.

Sure, tattoos can be cool—some are even beautiful. But they are forever, and as a mom, I just don't get it. What's a flower going to look like on eighty-year-old wrinkled skin, and what about in job interviews? My advice is, if you are going to get one, choose a spot that is pretty well hidden, at least at first. Wait until you are twenty years old, or go for a cute henna tattoo!

Yes, piercings are permanent, too. Even if you take out your nose ring, you are going to have a hole in the side of your nose for life. It is hard to realize when you are young that you are going to be any different than you are now, but you will be.

In general, I'm not a big fan of body piercing. Anyone who comes to see me for an interview with something in her or his tongue is an instant no. If I can see past it, I don't allow them to wear it to work. It is the motherly thing in me: why did you do that to such a gorgeous face? If you have to pierce something, at least do it in a place most people don't see. Remember, you will not always be seventeen.

nails

Nails are a great way to experiment without a lot of emotional or financial investment. You can raid the bargain bin at the drugstore or chemist for fun and funky colors that are in right this second (hello, black, silver, or orange nail polish).

I know a lot of girls love to grow their nails long, but I still like short nails the best. They are the most modern. It is all about being clean and well-manicured. If your nail polish is chipping, it doesn't look cool or punk. It's just messy. If you are going to paint your nails, make sure you have nail-polish remover and big cotton balls (much better than toilet paper) to take it off when your manicure is kicked.

For a really cutting-edge look that models sometimes wear backstage at the top fashion shows, give yourself a matte manicure. Apply nail polish without a topcoat. After it dries, run a nail buffer or chamois cloth over your nails.

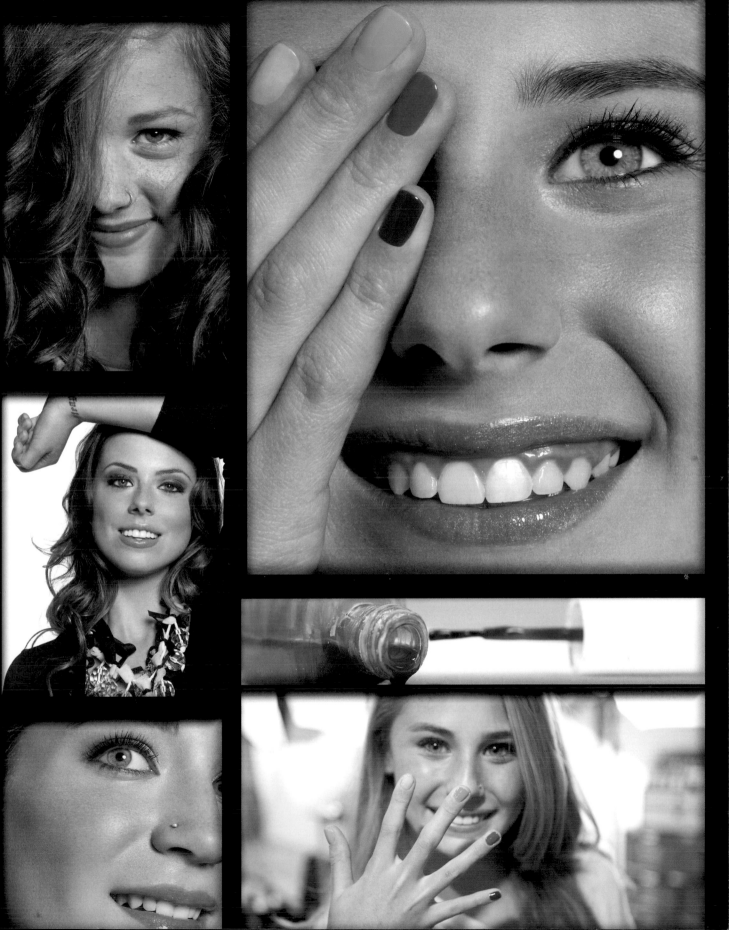

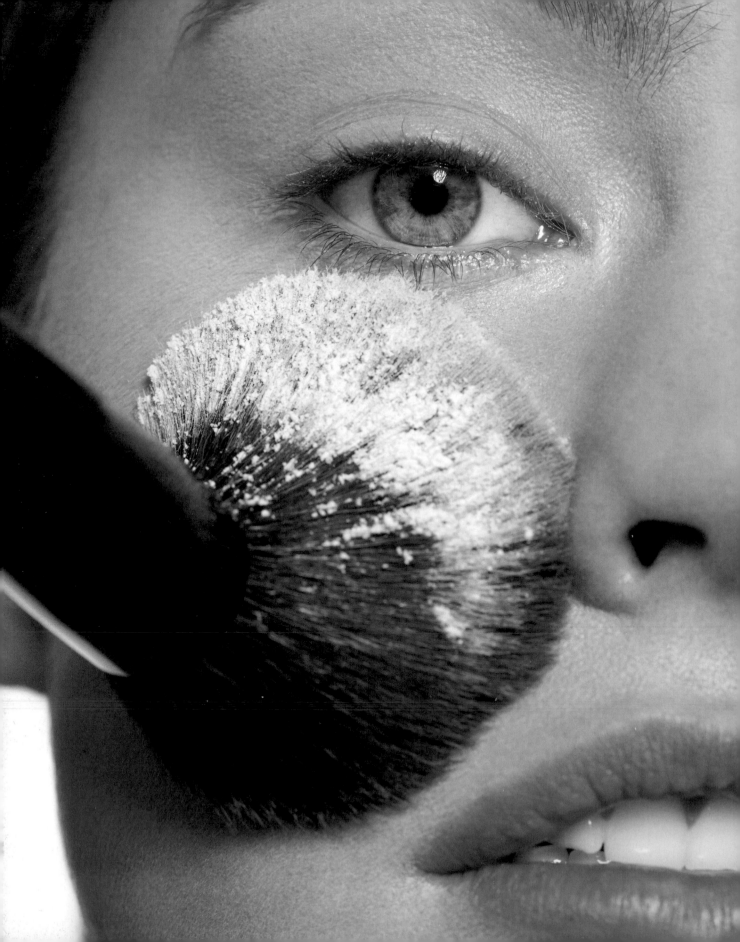

MAKEUP 101

I love makeup. From the product itself to the packaging to the way it looks, feels, and smells. Once I started playing with makeup, I never stopped. Now it's my world.

My mom let me put it on myself long before I wore anything out. My first memory with wearing makeup "out" was when I was about eleven or twelve. I still remember the compact that I used. Eye shadow only—in bright pastel color. Blue, green, lilac, pink, and peach. Matte color, not shiny. No sparkle. I remember applying it with my fingers, not a brush. And the mascara was matching. Yes, blue, green, or purple.

About this time I started going to parties, bar and bat mitzvahs, where it was okay to dress up and wear a little gloss, shadow, and a touch of blush (cream, as I remember). The great thing about being so young was that there was nothing to cover up (I was blessed with good skin). It was just about embellishing. I've learned a lot since then, but one thing hasn't changed: when it comes to makeup, young people only need to embellish to look amazing.

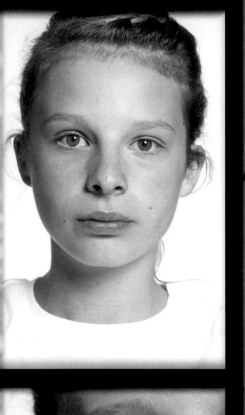
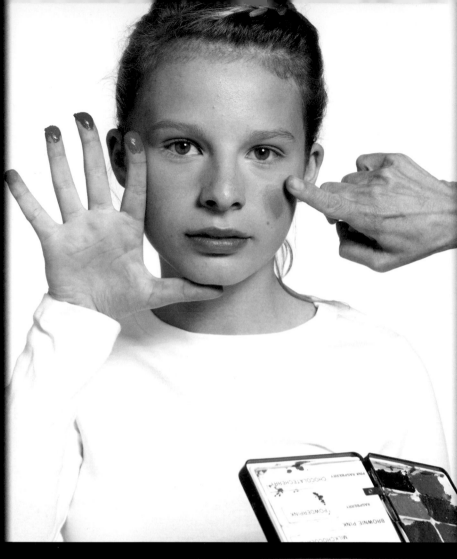
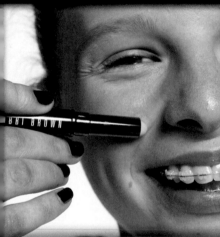
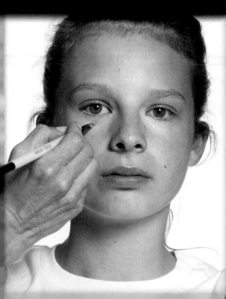
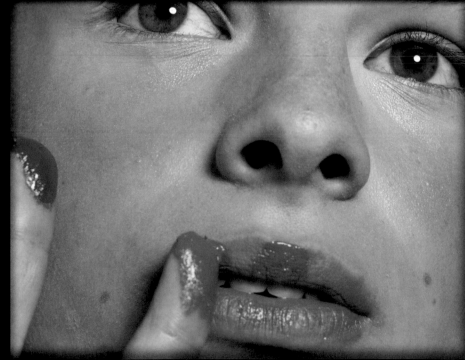

makeup in an instant

You have a lot going on in your life. School, friends, parents, sports, and the rest. That means there isn't a lot of time for putting on makeup. Still, you want to look your best. Somewhere between rolling out of bed, gobbling breakfast, and catching the bus, you can get pulled together with this easy five-minute basic makeover.

STEP 1: COVER PROBLEM SPOTS

Dab on foundation or blemish cover stick to cover any pimples (for more on pimples, see page 35) and concealer under your eyes as needed.

STEP 2: EVEN SKIN TONE

Use a tinted moisturizer with SPF all over your face. A light layer will even out your skin tone and provide necessary sun protection year-round (for more on skin tone, see chapter 7).

STEP 3: ADD COLOR

Rub a creamy blush on the apples of your cheeks. When you smile, the apples are the fleshiest part of your cheek. Blend up and down with your fingers (for more on blush, see pages 108–110).

STEP 4: ADD SHINE

Swipe lip gloss in a sheer color across your lips. If your lips are dry, opt for a tinted lip balm (for more on lips, see chapter 9).

STEP 5: DEFINE EYES (OPTIONAL)

Apply a coat of brown or black mascara to your lashes. If you have dark hair and naturally thick lashes, you can skip this step. Mascara goes on the top and bottom lashes. If you apply two coats, let it dry in between (for more on mascara, see page 120). I know some of you will also throw on eyeliner here, too.

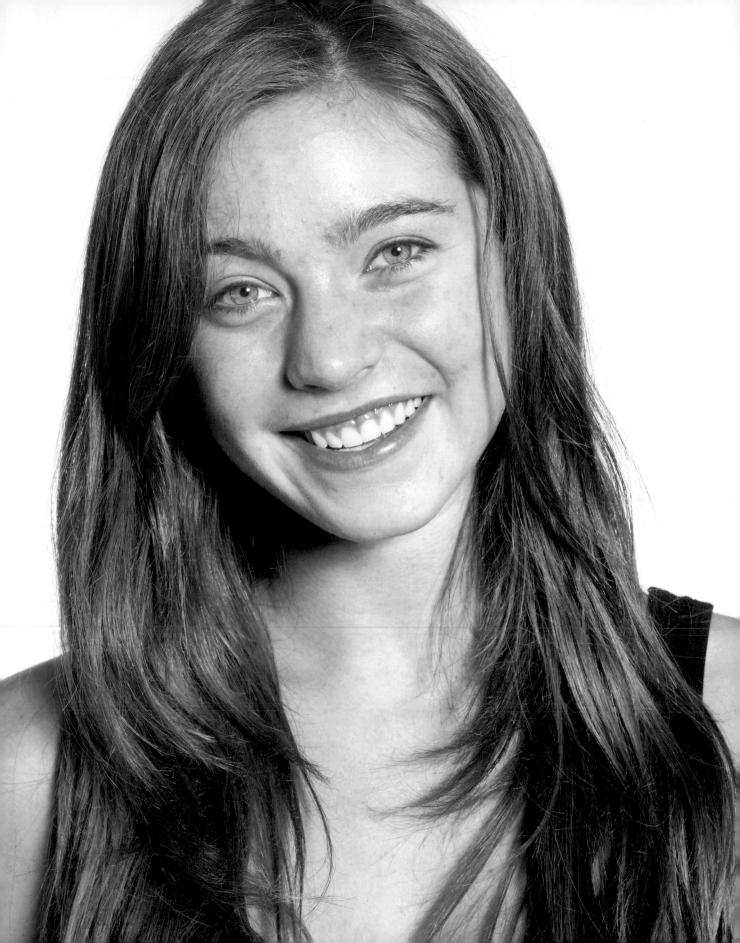

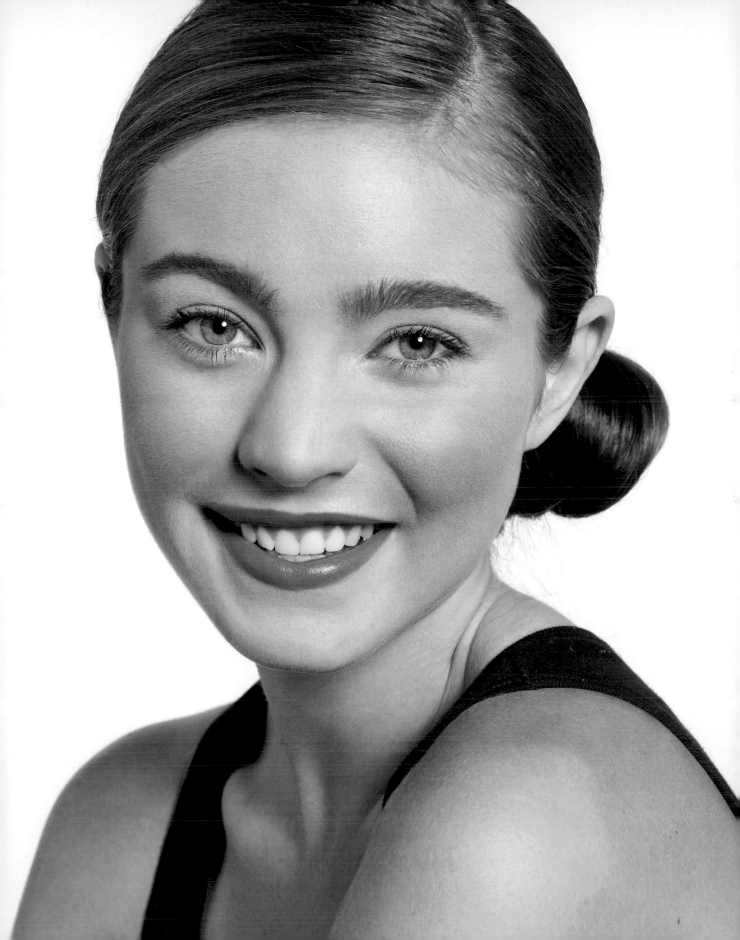

complete makeover

For a full makeup routine, follow these basic steps.

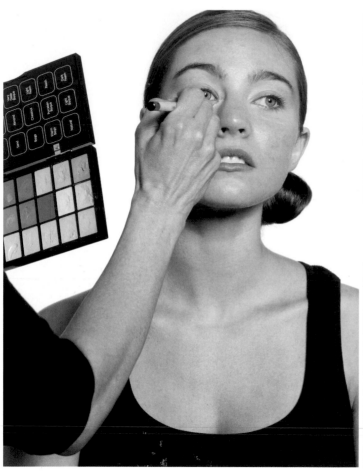 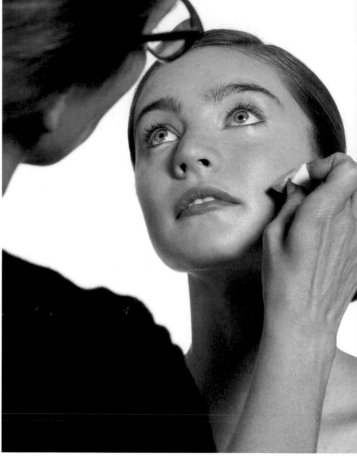

CONCEALER:

Layer a yellow-based concealer under the eye area, up to the lash line and inner corner of the eyes. If you use a brush to apply the concealer, blend by patting with your fingers. Finish up with a pale yellow powder to set the concealer in place.

FOUNDATION:

Use a brush, sponge, or your fingers to apply foundation wherever your skin needs it—which might be the entire face. There's usually a lot of redness around the mouth and nose.

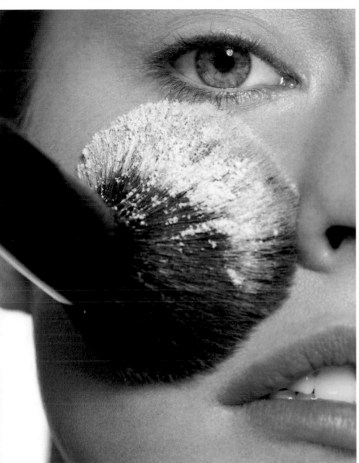

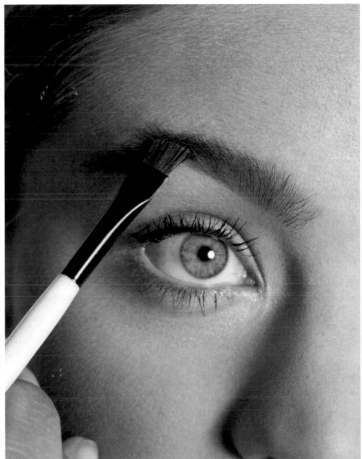

POWDER:

Apply loose powder where needed on the face, especially around the forehead, nose, and chin. For oilier skin, the powder goes all over.

BROWS:

Fill in your brows to add definition. Make short strokes with a shadow or eyebrow pencil that matches the color of your eyebrows and hair. For the most natural look, layer a powder shadow in a matching color on top.

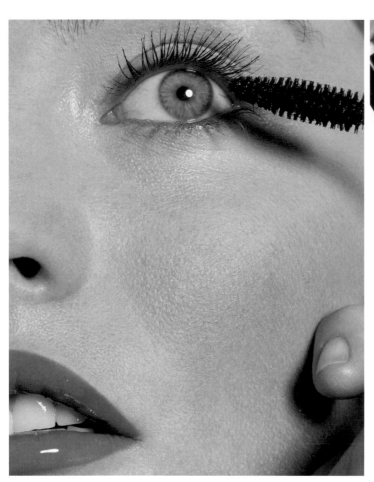

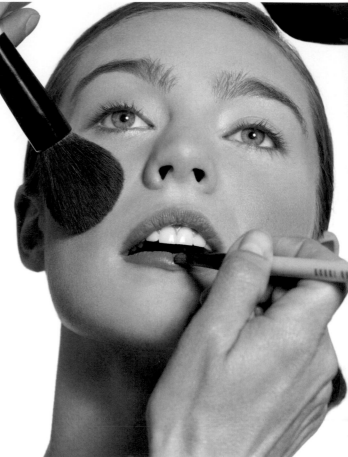

MASCARA:

Curl your lashes before applying mascara. Hold the mascara wand parallel to the floor. Brush lashes from the base to the tips while rolling the wand to avoid clumps. Let dry for a few seconds and repeat with second and third coats. (Optional eye shadow and liner steps: Apply a light eye shadow from the lash line to the brow bone. Follow with a stronger color on the lower lid. Line the upper lash line, making sure there are no gaps in color. If you line the lower lash line, make sure it is thinner than the top line.)

BLUSH:

Smile and apply blush to the apples of your cheeks, blending up toward the hairline and down toward the jawbone.

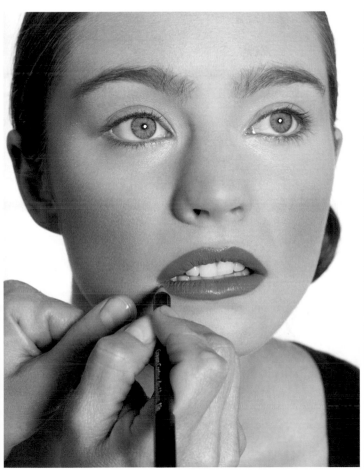 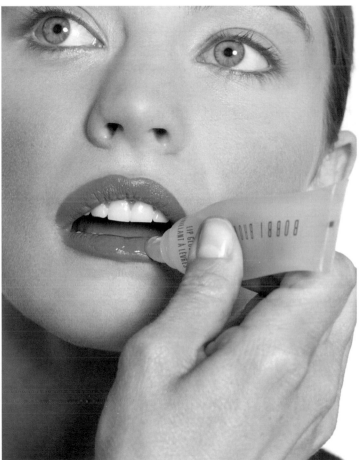

LIPSTICK:

Natural-looking lipsticks, sheer formulas, or glosses can be applied from the tube. But if you are using a very dark or bright color that needs to be precise, consider using a lip brush and lip pencil.

GLOSS:

A dab of gloss always creates a great shine. Choose a clear gloss when you don't want to change the color of the lipstick.

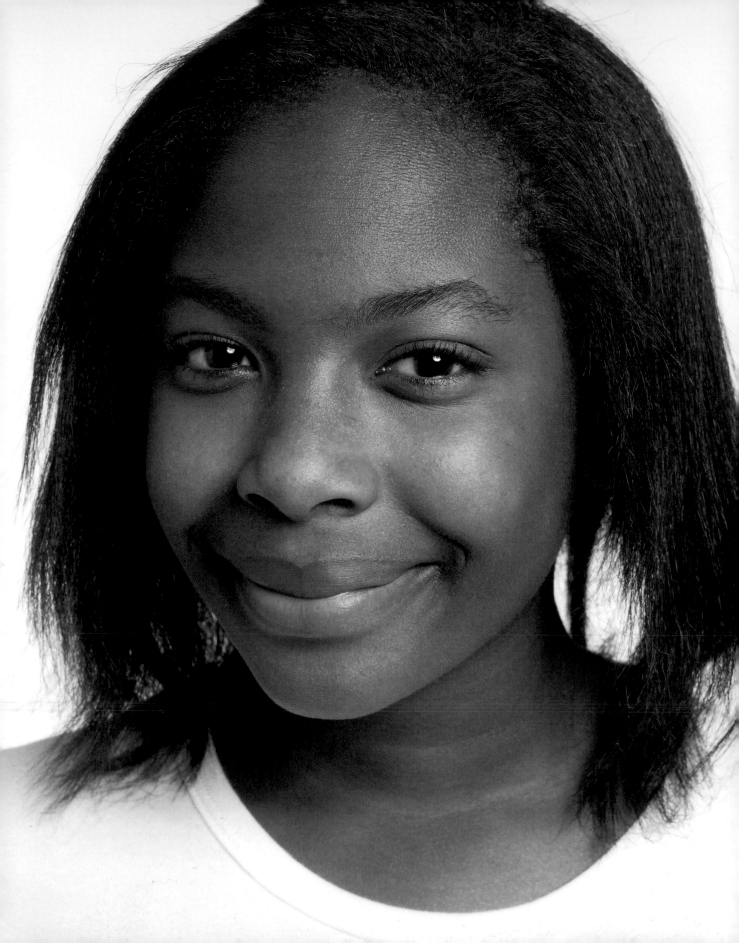

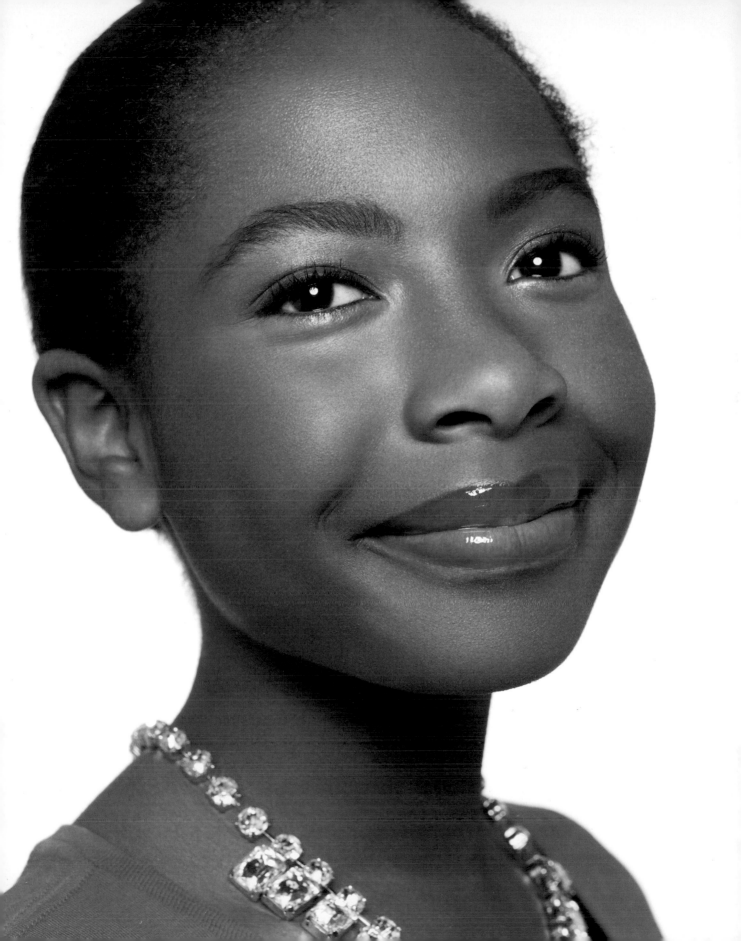

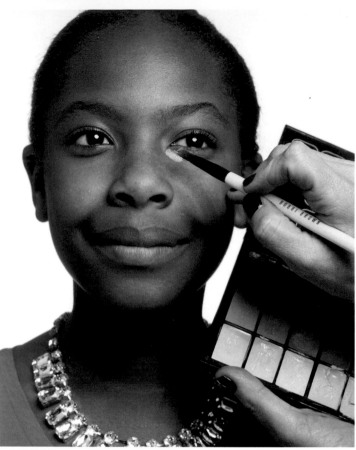

CONCEALER

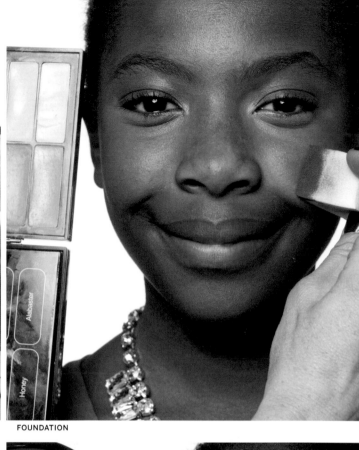

FOUNDATION

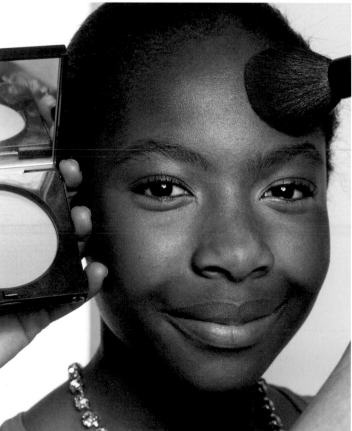

POWDER

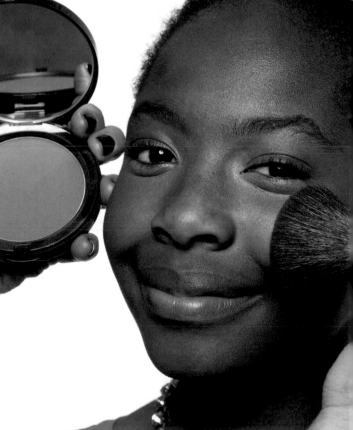

BRONZER

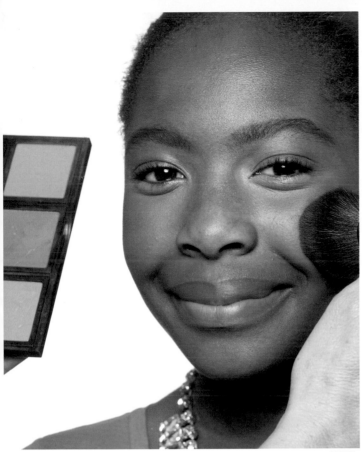

BLUSH

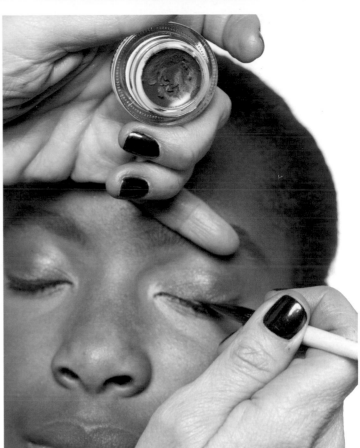

LINER

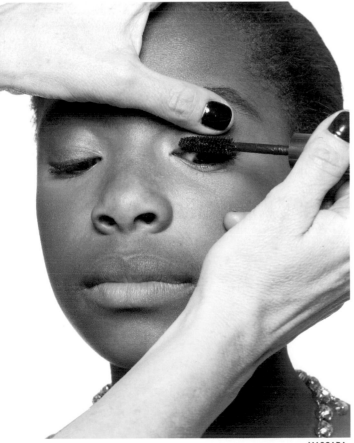

MASCARA

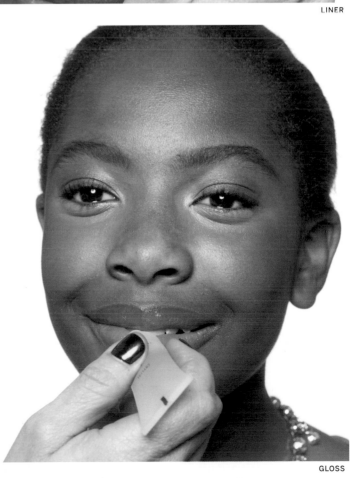

GLOSS

YOUR IDEAL MAKEUP KIT

There are so many beauty products out there on the market, it's crazy. Even though I own my own makeup line, I still love to shop for the stuff. The packaging is so cool, and all those colors! Still, makeup is expensive. Those little bottles can really add up. So it's good to know what you really need.

at home essentials

- Cleanser
- Eye makeup remover
- Tinted moisturizer with SPF
- Foundation or cover-up stick for covering up pimples
- Tweezers
- Brown or black mascara
- Eye shadow in one or two natural colors
- Eyeliner in powder, gel, or pencil
- Blush in a soft, natural tone
- Lip gloss or stain
- Lip balm
- Nail polish
- Nail-polish remover

fun extras

- Eyeliner, shadow, and nail polish in funky colors (don't spend a lot of money on these because they are just experimental)
- Eyelash curler
- Bronzer
- A set of makeup brushes
- All-over shimmer for eyes, cheeks, and lips
- False individual lashes or a natural lash strip

on the go

Keep it simple here. You're probably not going to give yourself a makeover in between classes, so why tote around a lot of unnecessary stuff? Plus, do you want everyone to see you fishing around for your lip gloss in a big bag of makeup? Throughout your day, carry these items in a small makeup bag or a pencil case.

- Cover-up stick to touch up pimples
- A small travel-size SPF for reapplication during warmer months
- Three-in-one pencil for lips, eyes, and cheeks
- Lip gloss, stain, or balm

INSIDE BOBBI'S BAGS

EVERYDAY BAG

In my everyday life, I try to carry as little as possible. Everything is getting slimmer, from phones to computers. Why shouldn't makeup? So I have created a super-stealth empty compact to fill with concealer, foundation, blush, lip stain, lip shimmer, and a matte lip color that fits in the palm of my hand. Even if I'm wearing a small purse for an evening out, my palette slides right in. That's for my own personal use.

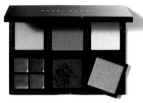

When I'm working, it's a whole different story. For photo shoots I lug around a professional kit that I have to hold in a suitcase it's so big.

PRO BAG
BY THE NUMBERS

46	39	120	60	40
BRUSHES	BLUSHES	EYE SHADOWS	LIP GLOSSES	LIP PENCILS

90	20	36	20
LIP COLORS	GEL LINERS	PALETTES OF MAKEUP	FOUNDATION SHADES

HERE'S A PEEK INSIDE (P.S. KIDS, DON'T TRY THIS AT HOME)

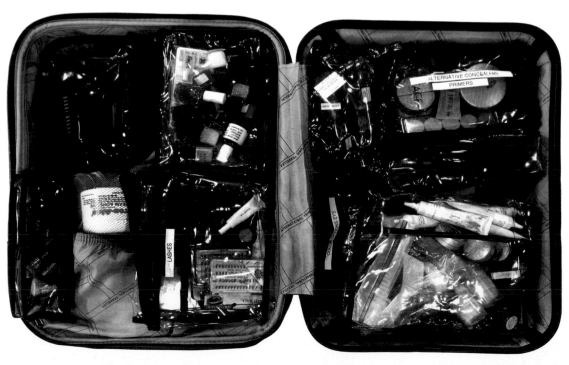

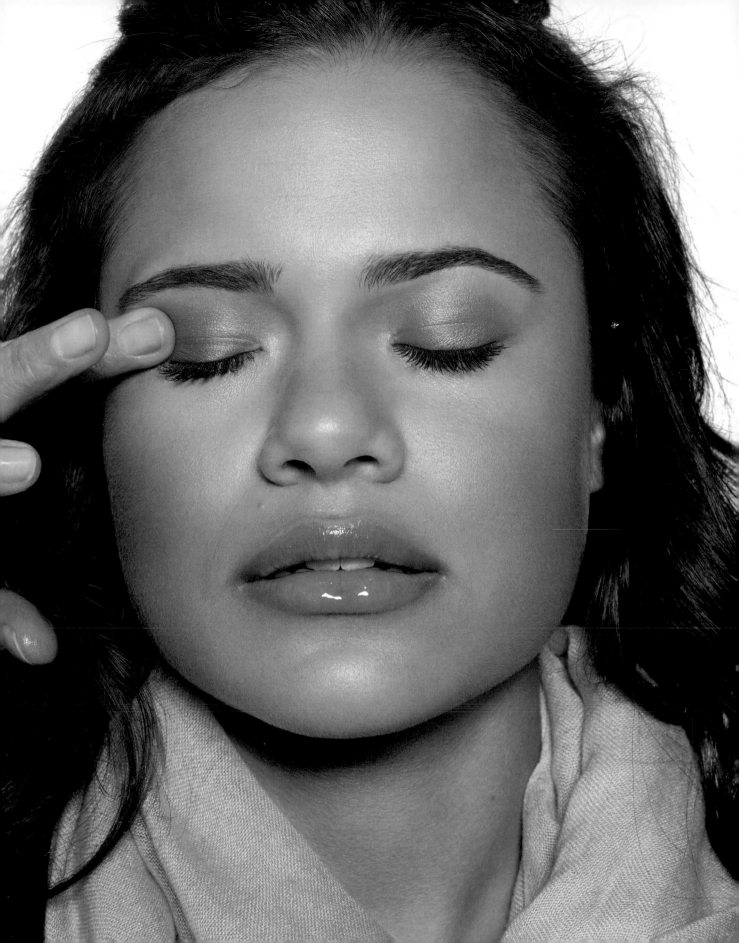

tricks of the trade

You might not be able to lug a makeup artist's kit around, but you can still act like a pro.

DO use your finger to apply makeup. Some salespeople at makeup counters will tell you this is the wrong move because it isn't as precise as using a brush, but I think they are wrong. Your finger is the best application tool around (except for eyeliner). The most modern looks are unfussy. Fingers are great for lip stains, cream blush, and shimmer. Have fun, experiment, and don't worry about being perfect.

DON'T throw out leftover lipstick or cream blush when there is so little product left that it's hard to get at in its original packaging (unless it's more than eighteen months old). Scoop the remainder out of the lipstick tube or blush compact into palettes you can buy at beauty- or art-supply stores. Write the name and color on the back of the palette in case you want to buy the product again.

DON'T use a magnifying mirror. You should apply your makeup as other people see it, not zoomed in for some crazy close-up. You won't get a good perspective on your look. Plus, when you see your pores magnified like that, it will tempt you to squeeze blackheads and other blemishes (i.e., pick your face), which is a really bad idea.

DON'T use makeup that's more than eighteen months old.

shop like a pro

There's a lot of makeup out there, and a lot of places to buy it. A girl can get overwhelmed easily. Here's the breakdown of the best places to shop.

DRUGSTORE OR CHEMIST

This is the place to stock up on all your basic beauty supplies, such as cotton balls, nail-polish remover, cotton swabs, and makeup sponges. Drugstores and chemists are really convenient and filled with bargains. The makeup is usually less expensive than in other kinds of stores, and often there are great sales. I love to shop the bargain bins for nail polish in crazy colors and other whim purchases. The only downside to this kind of shopping is that you can't test all the products before you buy them, so you might wind up being disappointed with the shade or texture.

DEPARTMENT STORE

Most high-end brands are sold at counters in department stores. This kind of makeup can get pretty pricey, but what you get in return is help from knowledgeable salespeople who are trained to put on makeup. These folks can give you lots of tips, ideas, and sometimes free samples (they also might try to pressure you into buying a bunch of things). Another plus is that you can try a product before you buy it.

BEAUTY SUPERSTORES

I love these one-stop shops because they have such a wide range of beauty products, from a totally classic fragrance to the craziest new false eyelashes. You can find mass-market makeup and niche products. The staff usually knows its stuff and can give you an objective answer about good products because the store isn't pushing any one line.

ART-SUPPLY STORE

Art-supply stores have always been a shopping resource for me. I like to buy the paintbrushes they sell to use as makeup brushes (for the shapes of the brushes, see page 111). They are a lot cheaper than the brushes sold at department or beauty stores and work just as well. You can also buy empty palettes for mixing your own lipstick colors or salvaging the leftovers from your favorite products.

WEB SITES

Once you know the products you like, nothing beats the convenience of shopping online. It's fast, easy, and you can do it when your homework's done. Browsing Web sites is also a good way of checking out the new colors, products, and looks offered by your favorite makeup companies.

tips when buying makeup

Makeup can be quite expensive, and there are so many choices. So be careful with your purchases. It's easy to get caught up in a sales pitch, returning home twenty dollars poorer with bright-pink lipstick you'll never wear in real life. Follow these tips to avoid the trap.

DO YOUR HOMEWORK

Make sure your basic products are up-to-date and still work. Then look for colors that catch your eye.

SHOP ON YOUR TIME

Try to hit makeup counters when they aren't crammed with shoppers. You'll get more attention from the salespeople and won't feel rushed in your purchases. The busiest times at department stores are lunchtime or weekends (unless you hit the store when it first opens).

FACE IT

Shop for makeup completely bare faced. That means not a stitch of makeup. You might feel self-conscious facing those painted ladies at the makeup counter au naturel, but it's the best way to tell if a shade works on you. A color should instantly enhance your natural coloring. My rule is, if you need other makeup to make a shade look good, don't buy it.

MAKEOVER MANIA

Doing makeovers is part of the business. Most companies offer free makeovers where you are under no obligation to make a single purchase (make sure to ask if you have to buy anything before the salesperson gets started). I know it can be uncomfortable after someone has spent thirty minutes working on your face to walk away empty-handed. But you shouldn't buy anything you don't love no matter what the salesperson says or how much she rolls her eyes. Just be polite. Thank them for their help and say you need to think it over.

LOOK FOR WHAT YOU LIKE

Makeup is like a lot of other things—music, clothes, friends. It's a matter of personal taste. If you want to get your makeup done at a counter, find a salesperson whose makeup you actually like. If you let a woman with old-lady pancake foundation and dark lip liner give you a makeover, guess what? That's what you're going to look like. Find someone who not only looks great but who is also nice. It's important to feel comfortable enough to say what you want to get from the experience.

SPEAK UP

Communication is the key! Tell the artist what you're looking for and what you like as she applies it. That will save you from having to go into the nearest bathroom to wash it all off!

FREEBIES

Ask for samples. Lots of companies are more than happy to let you try before you buy. Beware when buying products you can't try. Sometimes pink in the package looks pretty. But that same color can look like cake frosting or sunburn on the skin.

RETURN POLICY

Most large cosmetic companies will accept returns if you don't like a product, have a bad reaction, or find the packaging is damaged. Don't be shy about taking it back and explaining the problem. This stuff's expensive!

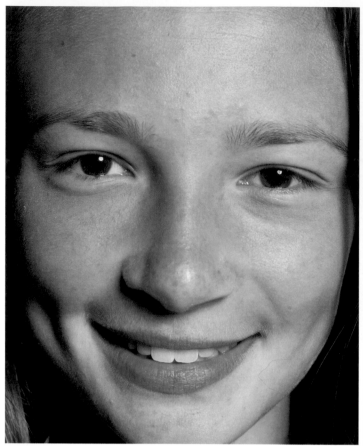

BEFORE

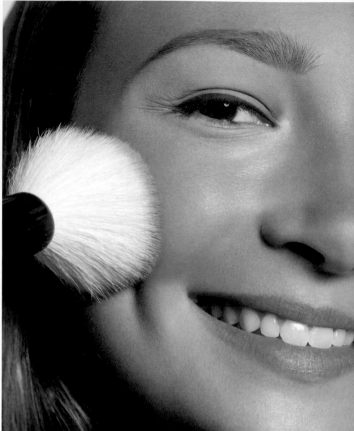

BLUSH

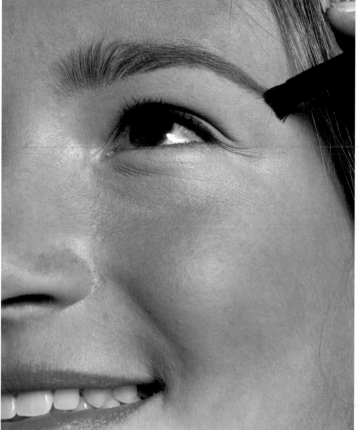

BROWS

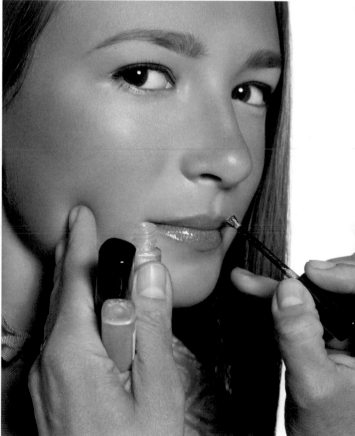

GLOSS

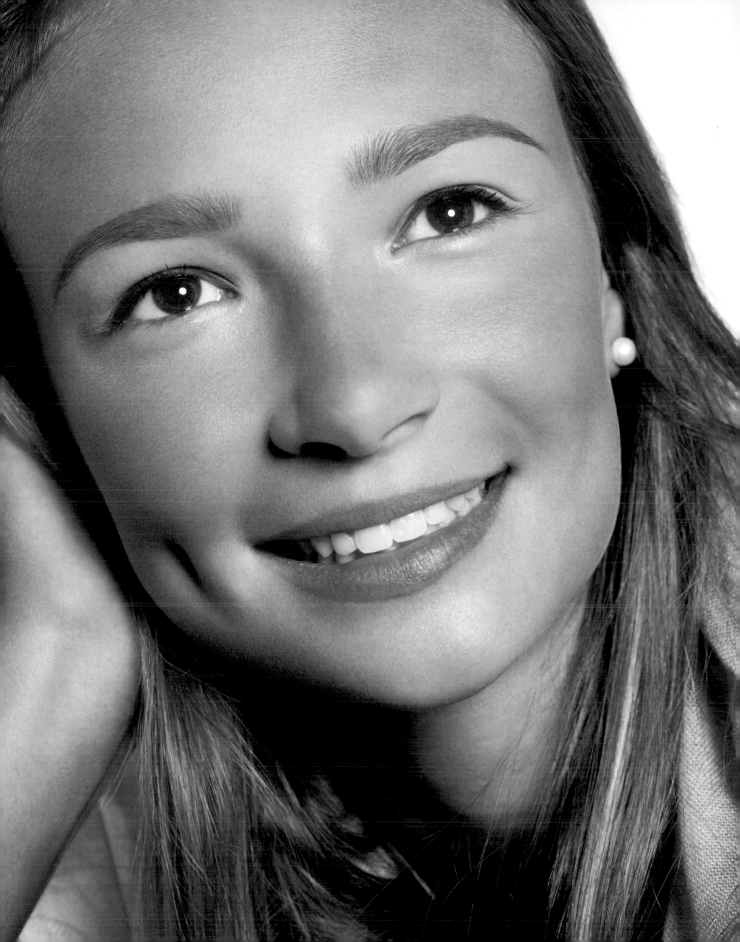

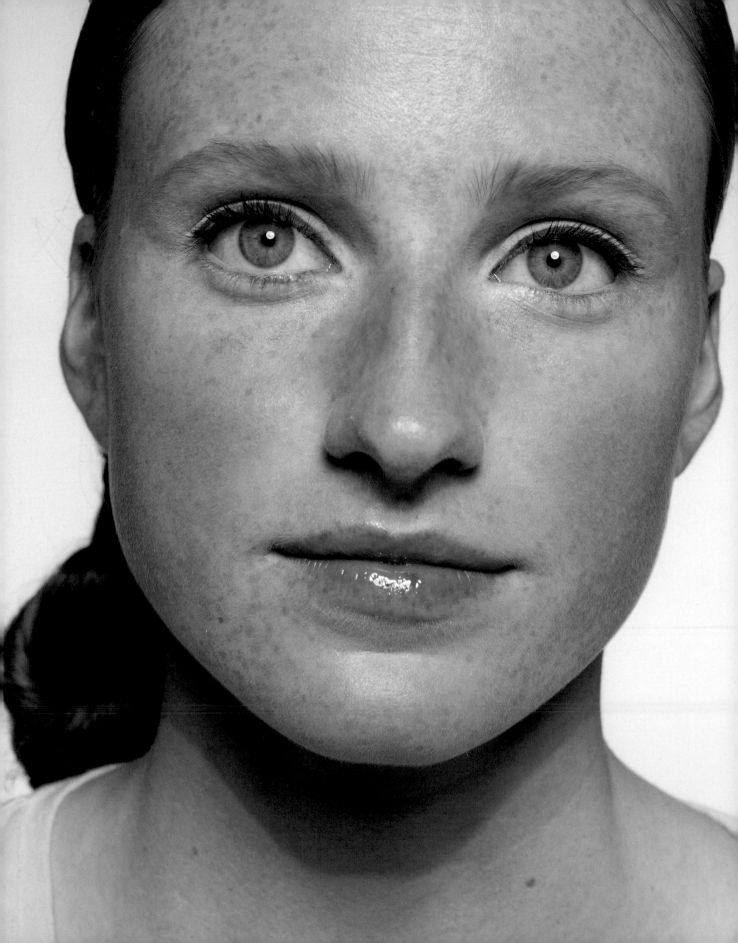

7

THE FACE

Evening out the skin tone in your face is the hardest and most important part of any makeup application. Getting it perfect is everything. The trick is to look like you aren't wearing any makeup at all. And that's all about matching your makeup to your skin tone.

The reason we wear concealer, foundation, and blush is to improve the way our skin looks. Everyone's skin is different, so the formula for getting that natural look will be unique to you. Some girls need foundation all over, some just a little concealer under the eyes, and some just need spot foundation to cover blemishes.

It is about having the right products and knowing how to use them so that your skin looks better. This isn't your mother's make-up. We aren't trying to hide under pancake. That's a mistake I see a lot of young women make. They buy foundation that they haven't tried and put on a thick layer to cover blemishes. The result? It looks like they are wearing a thick covering of makeup.

That's right; we actually want to see your skin. Once you learn how to even out the tone, remove the redness, erase the dark circles, and add color to your cheeks, you'll love what you see, too.

concealer

WHAT IT DOES

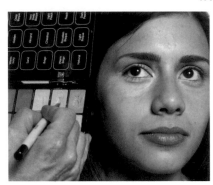

The name says it all. Concealers literally conceal things on your face or body. There are concealers that can hide anything, such as tattoos or scars, but the most common use is for lightening dark under-eye circles. The product should have a creamy texture for easy blending, and the tone is always lighter than the skin to create the brightening effect. Concealer is not for covering blemishes because the correct color for lightening dark circles will be too light to cover your pimple. It would actually make your blemish stick out. Apply concealer before you put on any other makeup because sometimes after you add concealer and brighten up the eyes, you don't even need foundation. You can wear concealer without foundation, but you can't wear foundation without concealer.

COLOR CHART

No matter what color you are—from very pale to dark brown—concealer should be one or two shades lighter than your skin. The product should also have yellow tones that help to lighten under the eyes.

HOW TO USE IT

Start with a sheer eye cream, especially if you have dry skin. Using a brush or your finger, apply the concealer under the eye starting at the inner corner of the eye. Cover the entire dark area below the lashes with the product and then blend by pressing it into the skin with your finger. Layer with a sheer yellow powder to lock the product in place and also to help blend it into the skin tone.

PRO TIP

If you don't need a lot of coverage, a stick foundation that's one or two shades lighter than the face can work as an under-eye concealer for those days when you wake up extra tired. If you are using regular concealer and it winds up looking too light on your face, warm up the area under your eye with a very light dusting of bronzing powder.

If you are extra dark under your eyes (sometimes with green or purple shades), try a corrector for more brightening. Corrector looks a lot like concealer, but this product brightens and lightens the area under the eye by correcting the color (concealer simply lightens the area). Use one with pinky tones for light to medium-light skin, and one with peach tones for medium-dark to dark skin. The corrector goes on first under the eye, starting with a brush on the deepest, darkest section and moving from the lash line down. Sometimes you need to apply more corrector than you would concealer, and even a second layer to correct the colors. After using corrector, you probably will need less concealer, if any at all.

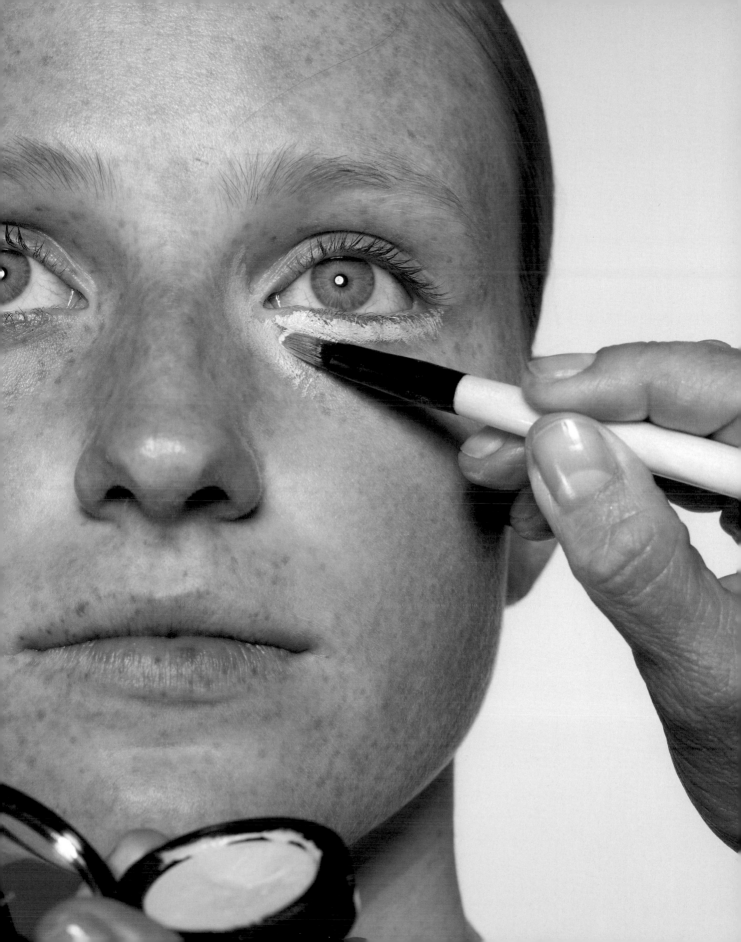

foundation

WHAT IT DOES

Foundation evens out the skin's tone and texture. It should be a natural tone and light texture because the end goal is clear and smooth skin. There are a lot of different formulas, including liquid, cream, and powder. For teens, I generally prefer tinted moisturizers because they are sheer and lightweight and often have the added value of SPF. You want your foundation to be diluted so that you can see your skin underneath. A denser stick foundation works for pimple coverage. A blemish cover stick is also great for covering the pimple and having it blend in to the skin tone.

COLOR CHART

Foundation in the right shade will disappear on the skin. The wrong shade will change the color of your face. You have to try different shades on your face to know which is the right one for you—preferably before you buy the product. At the store, cover a spot and look in a mirror that's near a window or a door. You will get the most accurate sense of how the color works on you if you can see it in natural light. If you see a little bit of pinkness on your skin, it's the wrong shade. There is nothing worse than looking like you applied a layer of calamine lotion to your face. Double-check the foundation color on your forehead, where the skin is sometimes darker. If it matches on the forehead, it will work everywhere.

FORMULAS

STICK is good for dry to medium skin.
LIQUID offers sheer to full coverage, depending on your skin type.
POWDER is only for oily skin.
TINTED MOISTURIZER is usually my go-to formula for great skin.

HOW TO USE IT

No matter what formula of foundation you use, your fingers are the best application tool. Your body temperature will warm up the product, making it easier to spread. Plus, you'll have the most control using your own hands (just make sure they are clean before you get started). You can also choose to use a sponge or foundation brush. Begin by applying a small amount of foundation around the nose (sometimes it's all that's needed). Then move outward, blending the foundation upward and into the hairline.

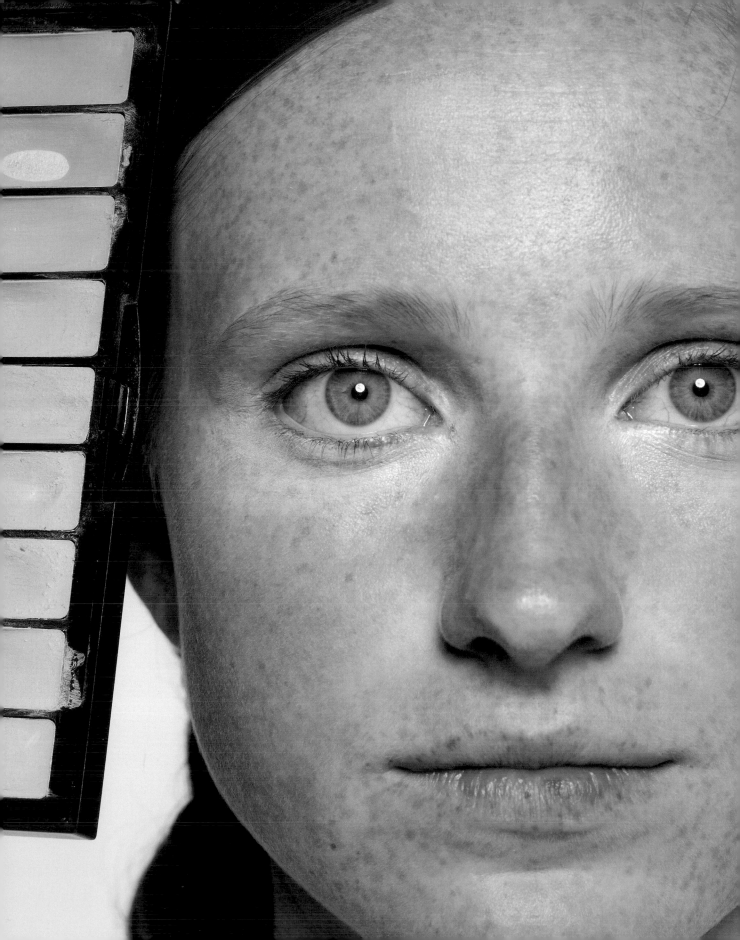

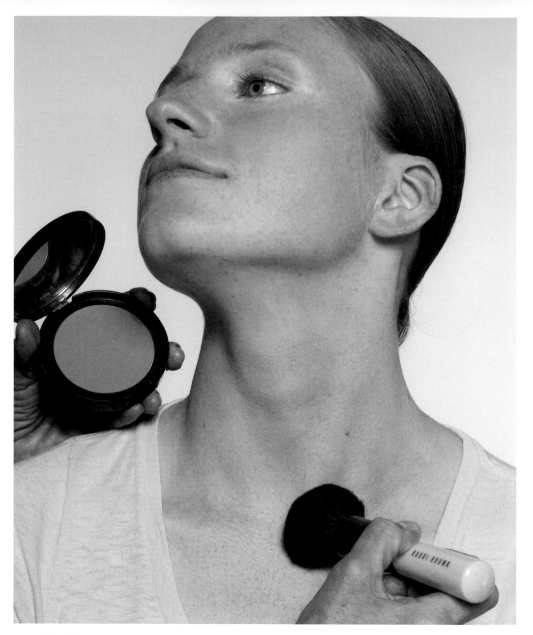

PRO TIP

Some people actually have more color in their face than their neck. If your face doesn't seem to match your neck (sometimes you are a bit darker on the face due to sun, irritation, and other things), brush your neck with a bronzer (for more on bronzer, see page 40).

I think every girl should own two foundations. You need one for winter months, when your skin is pale, and another for the summer, when you can't help but get slightly darker. You can mix the two foundations to create your own custom color for those times of the year when your skin is in between shades or to fix any areas of your face that are darker or lighter. You can also make your own tinted moisturizer: mix a bit of foundation with your favorite moisturizer in your hand, then apply to your face.

After you apply your overall foundation, use a blemish cover stick or foundation stick on any spots that don't have enough coverage.

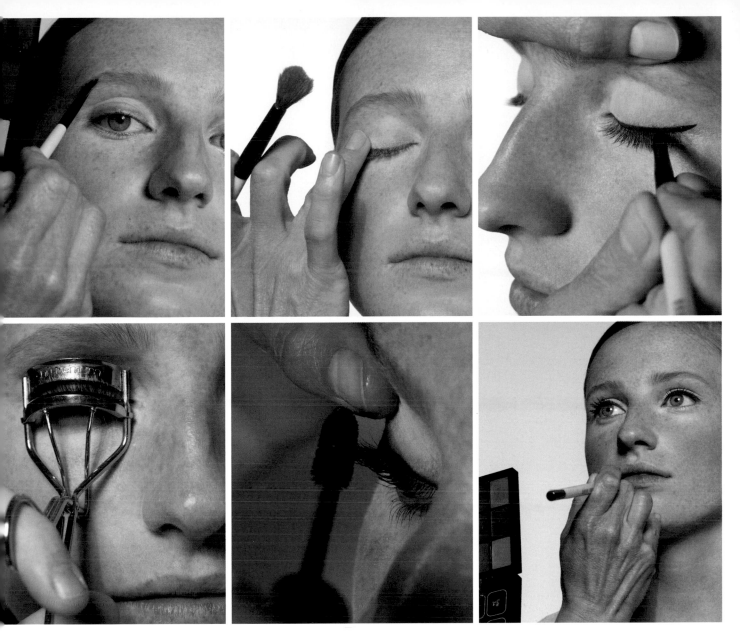

Because Hayley's neck is lighter
than her face, I brushed on a bronzer
to bring up the color (facing page).
To complement her freckles and
auburn hair, I filled in her brows
with a taupe color. Then, I added
a light shadow to her lids and a
brown eyeliner. I still like black
mascara for lighter lashes, and I
brought out the natural tones in
her lips with a warm pink (above).

blush

WHAT IT DOES

Blush makes you look fresh, pretty, and healthy. There are tons of blushes out there, so finding the right one for you can seem daunting. Go for the natural look, the one that says, "I've just had a great night's sleep and taken a fresh morning walk on a beautiful sunny beach." To replicate that healthy glow, check out the color of your cheeks right after you've had a good workout. That's the blush you're looking for. When you go to the store, remind yourself of the color by pinching your cheeks. Hold up different shades of blush next to your cheeks to see how they change the appearance of your skin, eyes, and even lips. You'll know the color isn't working if it looks too orange or if it makes your skin seem dull. When you hit upon the right shade, it will be, well, pretty.

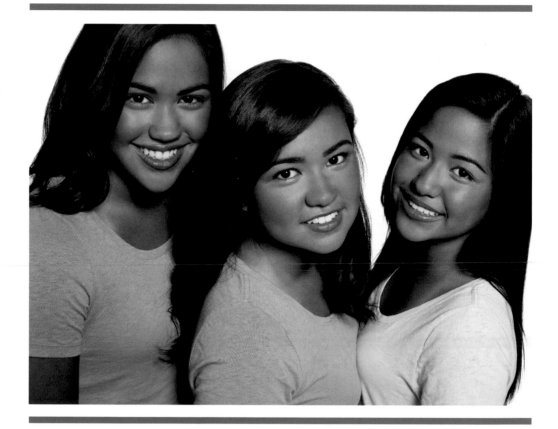

BLUSH TONES

The best way to find the right blush for you is to go shopping and check out how the colors look on your skin. But here are some basic rules of thumb to follow if you get confused.

SKIN TONE	BLUSH COLOR
VERY PALE:	Soft pastels without any brown tones, which would make skin look dirty
LIGHT:	Pale pink tones
MEDIUM:	Sandy pink to tawny tones
YELLOW OR OLIVE:	Rose or deep pink tones
DARK OR BLACK:	Soft plum or deep cranberry tones

BLUSH FORMULAS

Blush doesn't just come in many colors. There are also many formulas to suit different skin types and offer options when it comes to finishes.

POWDER:

By far the easiest and most mistake-proof formula. I recommend everyone have at least one powder blush because it works on all skin types.

GEL:

Gives a sheer color, but blending the gel to get an even tone on cheeks can be hard. This is best for totally smooth skin.

TINTS:

Similar to gel in that they offer sheer color but are usually in a stick form. They are a little easier to apply than gel but are still best for smooth skin.

CREAM:

Varies between denser and sheerer formulas. It's great for dry skin because it leaves a dewy finish after rubbed into the skin. However, it's not so great if you have breakouts. If you have covered blemishes with foundation, you will rub away your hard work when you apply the cream blush.

CHUBBY PENCILS:

The most portable blushes around. Pencils are easy to take with you throughout your day if you want to do your blush after school or touch it up at a party. These pencils do double duty and can also be used on the lips. They work best on normal skin. Dry skin sometimes makes them hard to blend.

HOW TO USE IT

Smile to find the apples of your cheeks, which are the fleshiest parts of your face. Apply the blush to the apples with a brush or your fingers.

Blend the blush up toward the hairline and down the cheeks to blend in with your skin.

Start slow and build the color. If you are using powder, blow a little off the brush before beginning so it doesn't stick. Layer one to two colors to get a pop on the cheek. If you are using your finger for creams, gels, or tints, dab lightly at first.

Stand back and bask in the glow of your beautiful cheeks.

PRO TIP

Blush fades in a few minutes, so applying two coats of either the same color or a brighter color on top, in the same formula, makes it last longer.

shop like a pro

For the best blush application, you need to get the right shape of brush. The skinny ones that come with the compact don't allow you to apply blush correctly; you need a full brush. If you don't want to fork over a ton of cash for a blush brush, head to my favorite beauty spot—the art-supply store—and get a soft, fluffy paintbrush.

It's important to take care of your brushes. To clean any brush with bristles, take a drop of gentle soap (like baby shampoo) into your palm, wet the brush, and swish the bristles in your palm to get them really soapy. Rinse thoroughly until all the soap is gone. Squeeze out the excess water with a clean towel, and reshape the brush head before you let it air-dry. Don't dry the brush on a towel because that can cause mildew to grow in the bristles. Instead, let the brush head hang off the side of a counter. Don't soak your brushes in water, either, because that will loosen the glue that holds the bristles and cause them to fall apart. If you clean your brushes every month or two, you'll really extend their life and save a lot of money.

YOUR BEST BRUSHES

There are hundreds of brushes out there. You don't need all of the basic ones below—some people start with a blush brush, others with an eyeliner brush. No matter which one you use, save up for quality brushes. They make a difference.

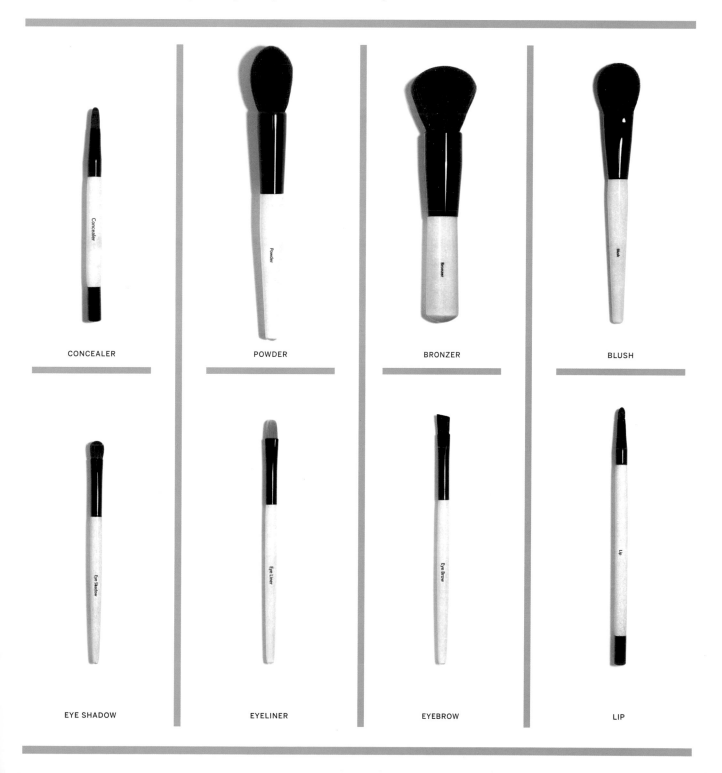

CONCEALER

POWDER

BRONZER

BLUSH

EYE SHADOW

EYELINER

EYEBROW

LIP

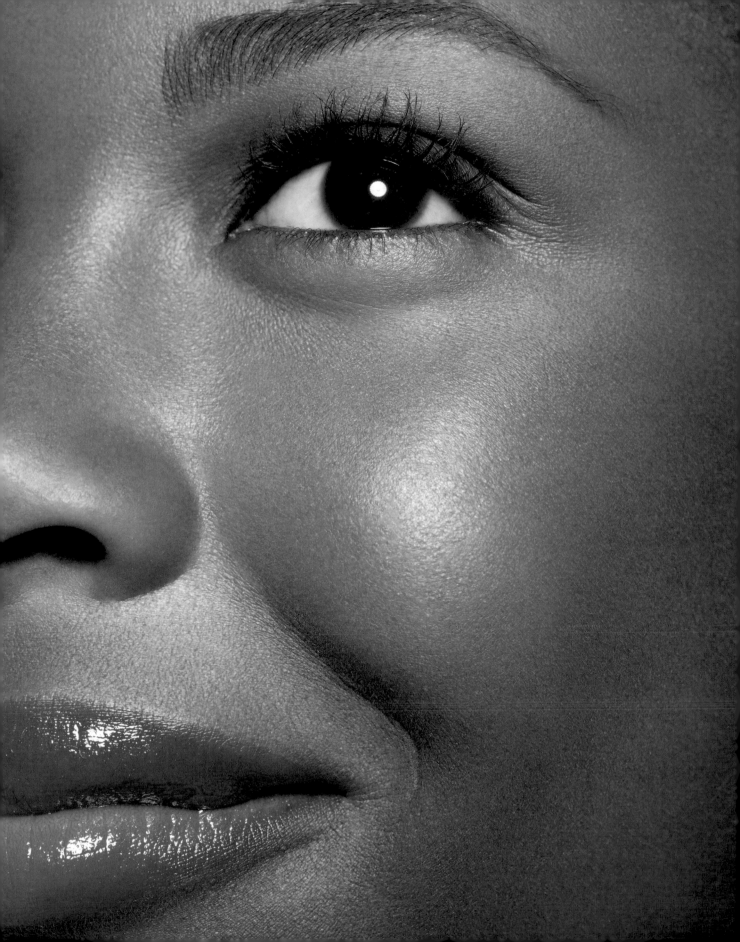

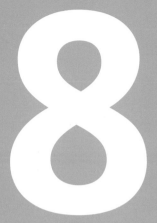

8

THE EYES

Clear, healthy, shining eyes. That's what I love, and that's what girls naturally have. You are filled with curiosity and energy, which is totally reflected in your eyes. No other feature outwardly expresses your inner beauty more than your eyes. You can use makeup to bring out that inherent sparkle. You can go really bold with eye makeup. Black liner is wildly popular with young girls, and it's a really strong option. But if your goal is to make your eyes pop, there are many different ways to go. So open your eyes to the possibilities.

eyeliner

Nothing is more important in making eyes pop than eyeliner. It defines their shape so eyes appear larger and more vibrant. When it comes to eyeliner, you can quickly have too much of a good thing. Master an artfully applied thin liner, and you will be amazed at how great it looks. Here's what you need to know.

EYELINER FORMULAS

GEL AND LIQUID: These are the bad boys of eyeliner. Even though they are the most difficult to apply, with practice, it's a breeze. You will need a rock-steady hand. One tiny shake or mistake and it shows. But the accuracy they provide is amazing for dramatic looks. Plus, these are long-wearing, smudge-proof, and water-resistant formulas. Try applying these liners at home when you aren't in a rush or under pressure to get somewhere. The more you practice, the better you'll get at it.

PENCIL: This is the easiest kind of eyeliner to apply (you started playing with colored pencils when you were a kid, right?). But, unfortunately, they smudge just as easily. If you are loving the pencil, set your eyeliner with eye shadow or powder after you've applied it to your eyes—this will help it last longer.

SHADOW: This technique is easier to apply and it gives a softer effect, but it's not as long lasting as gel. Shadows are great for creating a smoky eye and soft lines. To apply a shadow correctly, you'll need an eyeliner brush that's thin, stiff, and flat. You can either apply the shadow dry, or dip the brush in a little water and then into the shadow for more defined, denser color that will last longer than powder alone. Shadow can also be applied over a gel liner to soften the effect. (For more on smoky eyes, see page 232).

APPLICATION TIPS

Start with a thin line at the inner corner of the eye and gradually thicken the line as you move to the outer corner (I sometimes start from the outside and gradually thin it as I go in). It wakes up your whole face.

Use liner only on the top lash line to create a really pretty, clean look. This is key for big and beautiful looking eyes. If you also use eyeliner under your eye, keep it thin and smudged close to the lash line. The lower line should always be thinner than the top lash line. Otherwise it will draw more attention to under the eye and make you look tired. And please don't ever line just the lower lash line.

Liner inside the eye can look very rock star, but it does two things—it makes your eyes look smaller, and it always gathers in the corners.

Make sure there is no gap between your liner and lash line. You can apply more eye shadow with an eyeliner brush, which is a stiff, small brush, to fill in any spaces left by your liner. Your lashes will look crazy thick.

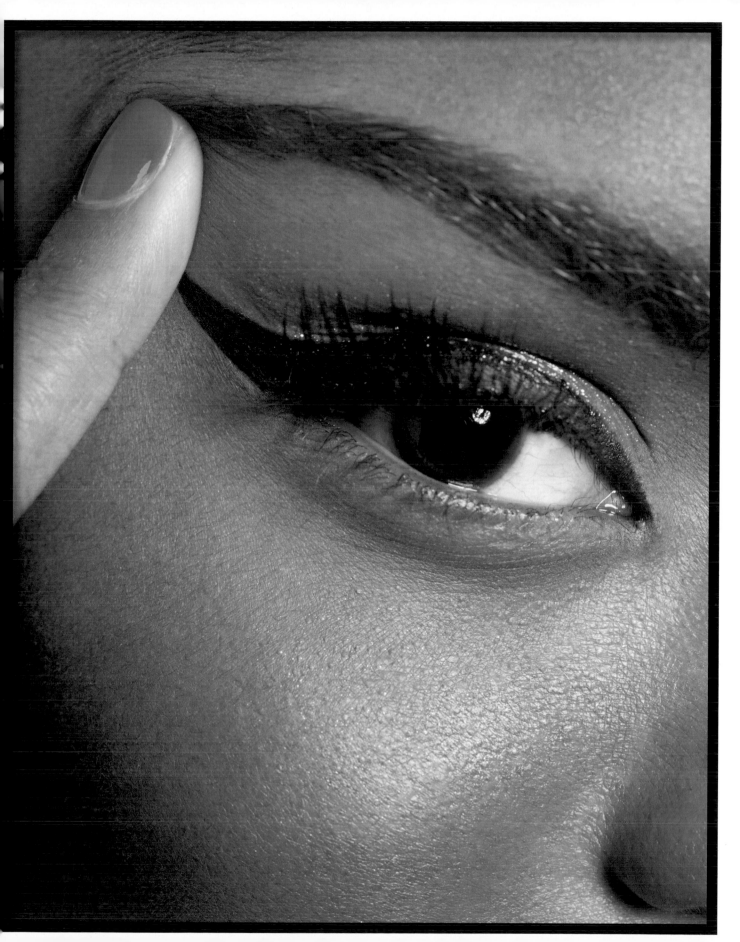

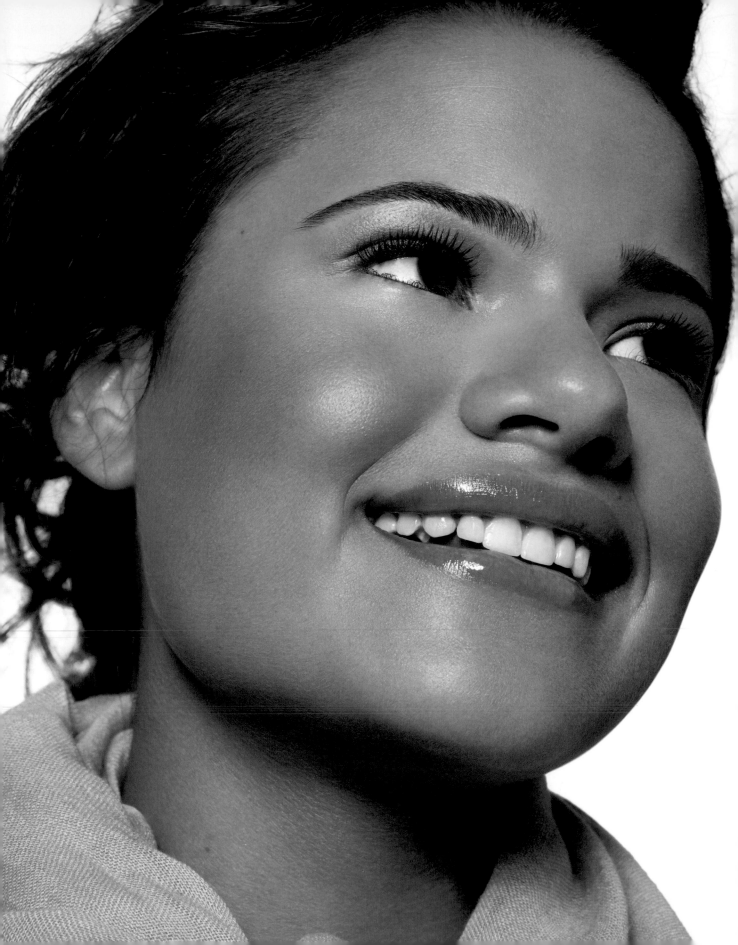

Black liner is a classic. I know girls love it and will wear it everywhere (I've even seen them wear it hiking). Just know that black is strong and gets stronger the more you put on. Also, you must wear concealer with black liner or it makes your circles look way darker.

eye shadow

It's great to experiment with neutrals, pastels, and metallics on your lids. You can also experiment with formulas such as powder, cream, or pencil. Don't worry about being perfect. Just spread a shade across your lid and see how it looks. Here are a few things to keep in mind.

If you have oily eyelids or are doing special makeup that needs to last through a long event, dust your lids with face powder before applying eye shadow. This creates a base for the shadow to stick to.

If you're using powder shadow, do your eyes and concealer first, and clean up any messes with a non-oily makeup remover and cotton swabs before you move on to the rest of your face.

Cream shadows come in formulas with and without powder. If you use one without powder in it, first apply a base powder to the eyelid and then follow with the cream shadow.

SHADOW TONE CHART

There are some eye-shadow colors that work with most eye colors—they include champagne, icy platinum, ash, and taupe. Here are some alternate shades to complement your eyes.

EYE COLOR	SHADOW COLOR
BLUE:	Blue in colors lighter than your eyes, heather, and lilac
GREEN:	Icy greens and heather
BROWN:	All browns

For most days, go for natural-looking shadows that complement your eye color. Leave the bright blues, brash purples, and other statement hues for special occasions.

Looking for a surefire way to get glam? Try a light and sparkly eye-shadow color like white, platinum, or gunmetal. Then sweep black liner onto your top lash line, and you're ready to rock. (For more smoky eyes, see page 232.)

brows

Eyebrows are the unsung heroes of the face. Sure, eyes get all the compliments. But brows that are shaped and groomed well are sophisticated, polished, and sexy.

The natural shape of your eyebrows is most likely the best for your face. Sometimes all it takes is to clean up between the brows. Then simply brush brows into place with a clear brow groomer for an instantly neater look.

If your brows are really unruly, go to a professional, who can create a natural-looking shape that works with your face. Even if you don't have especially heavy brows, shaping them can give you a much cleaner look. Tweezing is the best method of hair removal because it is quick and precise. Have the pro clean up the dreaded unibrow—the area in between the brows—and follow your natural arch.

After you've had your brows done, maintain them yourself with weekly or biweekly clean-ups, using tweezers with a flat, angled tip. Plucking right after you come out of the shower, when the skin's pores are open, will be less painful. Good lighting is a must. If you find any ingrown hairs, don't pick at them. Exfoliate the brow with a grainy scrub.

Filling in your brows with eyebrow pencil or shadow is another great way to add definition. First, set any unruly hairs in place with an eyebrow brush. Then shape brows or fill in sparse areas with an eye pencil or shadow that matches the color of your eyebrows or hair. If you use a pencil, try layering a little shadow on top for a softer, natural look. To apply the product, begin at the inner corner of the brow and follow its natural shape using light, feathery strokes.

Note to Parents: It's very common for girls to attack their brows at a sleep-over or overnight camp—often resulting in the dreaded tadpole brow. So if your daughter complains about her brows, take her to a professional, and instruct that person to go slow!

STRONG BROWS MAKE A BOLD AND BEAUTIFUL STATEMENT.

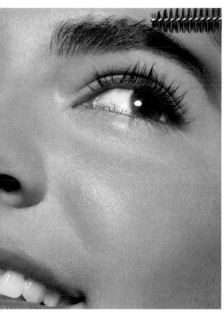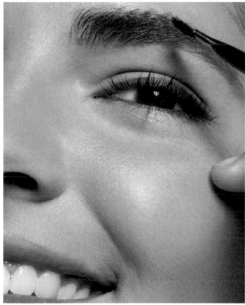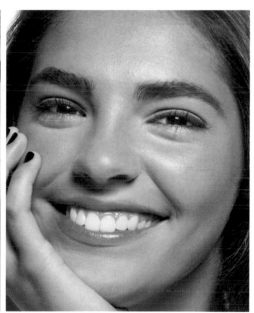

Embrace your strong brows if you have them. I honestly wish I had the brows I did in high school, before I went to town with the tweezers. With full brows, sometimes I just brush them up with a clean mascara wand. You can also add a little bit of definition with a shadow or pencil—make sure to use a natural color for a super-polished look.

mascara

Sometimes all it takes is a couple of coats of mascara to feel like you're ready to face the world. Black mascara is my weapon of choice because it helps all eyes stand out the best.

The first step is to curl the lashes. Or not. It's a lash saver if your lashes stick straight out. Make sure the lashes are always mascara-free before you curl; otherwise, they will break. If you have an eyelash curler, hold your hand up and away while you press down at the base of the lashes for five to ten seconds. Then apply mascara. No curler? No problem. Gently curl your eyelashes up with your finger as your mascara dries.

Don't pump the mascara wand in the tube. This sends air into the bottle and will dry out the mascara. Before you apply the product, blot the end of the brush with a tissue to get rid of clumps and excess mascara.

Apply the mascara under your top lashes, from the base up to the tip, holding the wand parallel to the floor and rolling it as you go to separate lashes. Mascara never goes on the topside of your upper lashes or it makes them droop. Let it dry if you are going to also do the bottom lashes.

Coats count. For maximum drama with your mascara, be sure to do two or three coats on your lashes. To prevent clumping, allow mascara to dry for a second or two in between coats. You can also use wands without any product or an eyebrow brush to separate the lashes after you apply the mascara. Inexpensive wands are sold at beauty stores.

Waterproof mascara is good when it's really hot and humid out or you're planning on shedding a few tears (weddings, breakups, anyone?). You need to use eye-makeup remover to take it off.

Colored mascaras are fun when you want to make a statement. Just make sure the tones are dark. Try navy, wine, or even ivy.

QUICK TIPS FOR AMAZING EYES

TIP NUMBER 1:
LAW OF PROPORTION

WHEN IT COMES TO EYELINER, THE LOWER LASH LINE SHOULD ALWAYS BE THINNER THAN THE LINER ON THE TOP LASH LINE. YOU DON'T WANT TO DRAW ATTENTION TO THE AREA UNDER YOUR EYE.

TIP NO. 3: MAKE IT STICK

DUST EYELIDS WITH FACE POWDER BEFORE APPLYING EYE SHADOW FOR LONG-LASTING WEAR.

TIP NUMBER FIVE: TONE IT DOWN

After you fill in your brows with a pencil or shadow, if the color winds up looking too harsh, soften it by pressing loose powder onto the brows with a powder puff.

TIP NO. TWO: LIGHTEN UP

Always wear concealer when you use black eyeliner. Otherwise, you'll wind up looking tired.

TIP NUMBER 4: BREAKING POINT

ALWAYS CURL YOUR LASHES BEFORE YOU APPLY MASCARA SO YOU DON'T DAMAGE YOUR LASHES.

WHETHER THE LOOK IS SIMPLE OR STRONG, LET YOUR EYES STAND OUT.

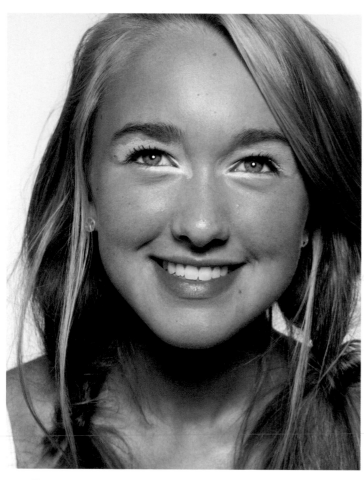

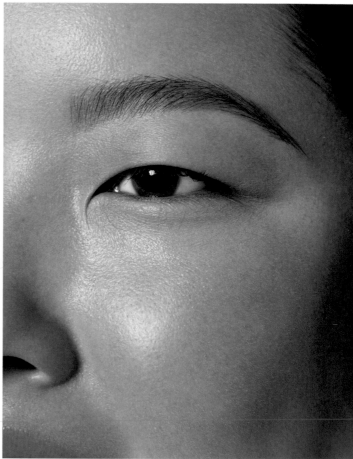

If you are going to experiment with color, do something fun and different. But make sure the rest of the face is pretty. Here, I used a light-green shadow and a little bit of white underneath the eye, topped with an ivy-colored eyeliner and black mascara. The rest of the face is neutral. It's fun, but she still looks good.

This look proves that you don't always have to wear eye shadow to get incredible eyes. Some liner, mascara, and an artfully filled-in brow create a beautifully polished appearance.

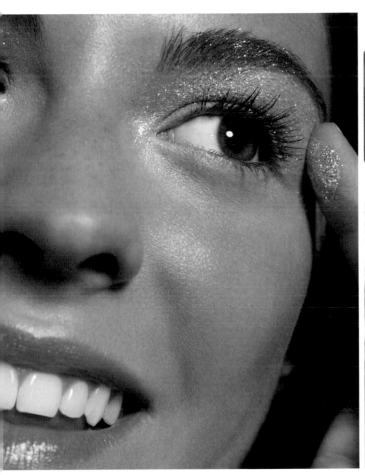 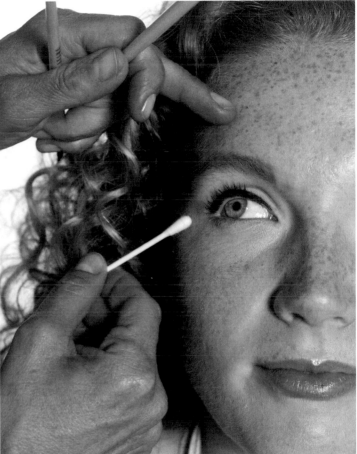

Playing with shimmer and glimmer is a great way to make a statement. Apply gold sparkly eye shadow over the lids and up to the brows. Use your fingers to get a denser application—the more shadow you get on your lids, the more they'll sparkle.

Black eyeliner makes blue eyes pop. Always have a cotton swab on hand to get rid of any smudges. First use a dry cotton swab. If there are still leftover smudges, wipe them away with a swab dipped in eye-makeup remover.

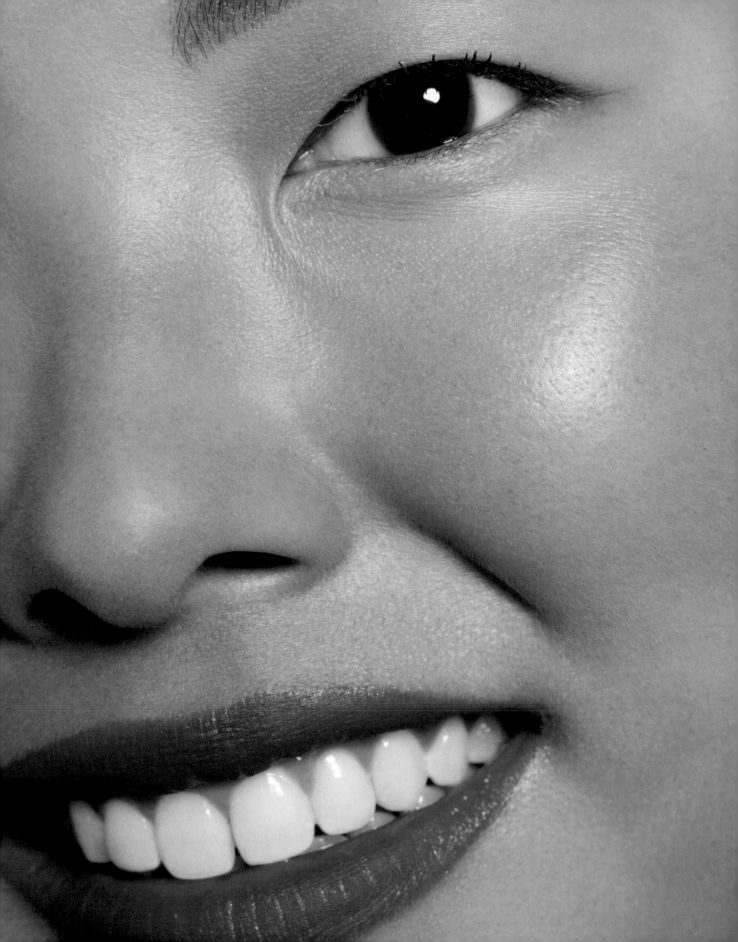

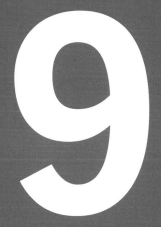

THE LIPS

There's nothing easier than a sheer lip color to make you look pretty. You can start with a clear gloss or balm, which is subtle and beautiful. If you are ready to move on, add a little bit of sparkle to your gloss. The shine will totally change your look. For girls, matte lips aren't necessary. Dark, matte lipstick will create a really strong mouth and will make you look older. For young, gorgeous lips, I'm more a fan of sheer pinks and berry stains, which are so modern and mistake proof. But go ahead, try it all and see what's best for your smile.

lipstick formulas

There are lots of choices when it comes to your lips. I love sheer colors and stains because they are easy to use and look gorgeous. Here are some other choices.

MATTE lasts longer than other formulas because it has more pigment, which helps it stick to the lips. The problem is that this dense product can dry lips out quickly and is often just too strong for some girls.

SEMI-MATTE has more moisture than a true matte, so it is good if your lips are dry, and it has a soft sheen that looks pretty.

LIP GLOSS gives lips lots of hydration. It offers a lot of shine, which makes lips look fuller. I like it on its own or layered on top of other lip colors. Lip gloss comes in sheer color or full color, with or without glitter and shimmer.

BALMS are made from formulas that specifically soften or heal dry lips. They come in clear and tinted varieties. They can also have sunscreen. It's pretty hard to make a mistake with these.

STAINS offer long-lasting, rich color that penetrates the lip.

CHUBBY LIP PENCILS can be used to define the lips and color them in. They have a creamy matte or sheer texture that lasts a long time.

LIP LINERS are generally used to define the lips and work as a base coat on the entire lip area so that lipstick or gloss on top of them lasts longer.

made in the shade

When you are shopping for that perfect lipstick—you know, that go-to tube you always keep in your bag—let your lips be the guide.

I have found that lipstick colors one or two shades darker than your natural lip color are the most flattering. They are also mistake proof (no chalky red lips or goopy white gloss here).

Go shopping for lipstick with no makeup on and take a good look at your lips. Then find a shade that looks similar to what you see but a bit deeper.

You know you've hit gold, or the right shade, when it makes your face and eyes look brighter without a stitch of any other kind of makeup. Pow! That's the power of lipstick.

Once you've found a perfect neutral shade for you, it's a good guide for going darker or lighter (but don't go more than one tone lighter than your natural lip color, or your lips will take on a creepy grayish, ashy look). Your shade will still be the basis for more dramatic colors.

LIPSTICK SHADE CHART

Just like with blush, foundation, and lots of other products, the best way for you to find a great gloss, stain, or lipstick is to observe your own lip and skin color. Try out a lot of colors until you get it right. But here are some basic guidelines.

LIP COLOR	LIPSTICK COLOR
PALE:	Beige, pale pinks, and light corals
MEDIUM:	Brown-based shades of rose, mauve, and berry
DARK:	Deep plum, chocolate, and red

PRO TIP

Some very fair women have almost blue or red lip color, so pale shades look too ashy. And many dark-skin-toned girls have the most beautiful pale pink lip color.

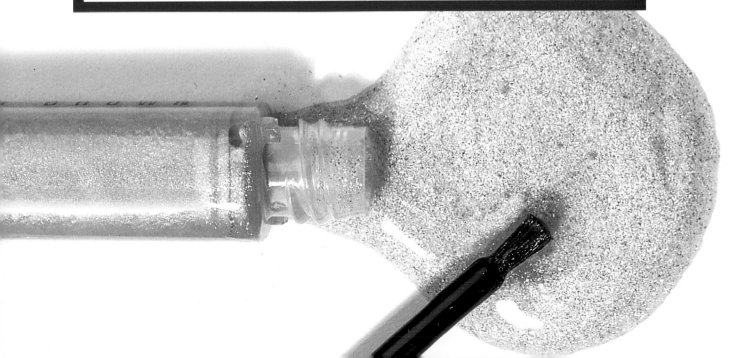

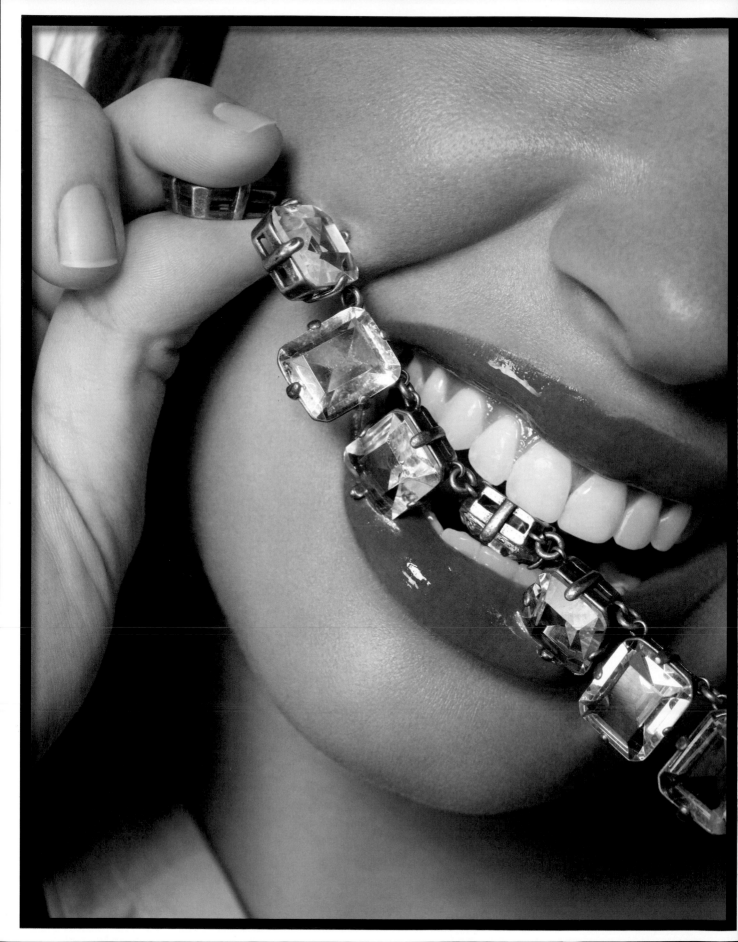

tricks of the trade

MIX MASTER

Channel your inner makeup artist. If you want to play like the pros, blend the colors from different products right on the back of your hand using a lip brush. If that seems too complicated, you can just use your finger and mix the colors directly on your lips. It doesn't matter if you start the mixture with a lighter or darker shade. If the color comes out too intense, mix in a little beige, which will mellow it out. But stay away from white, which makes colors look pasty. You can also mix textures to create your own glossy stain or shimmery gloss.

STAINPROOF

As I said, I love stains. The colors are so easy to put on you don't need a mirror. Stains are super-cool and modern. But you don't have to buy a separate product to get the look of a stain. Make a do-it-yourself stain by applying a really dark, bold, or bright shade and then blotting most of it off.

LIP-SMACKING LONG

I'm not a big fan of products that call themselves "long lasting" because often they are so dry, they'll turn your lips into leather. Instead, use a lip pencil as a primer for your lip product. Before you put on lipstick, apply a lip pencil that matches your natural color by completely filling in the lips. Then apply your lipstick, which will cling to the layer of pencil. You can also use a pencil that matches your lipstick after you've applied your lipstick to seal in the color. If you don't have a lip pencil, take a little bit of powder or blush and pat it over your lipstick. Add a bit of balm or gloss on top to remoisturize. Any of these methods will keep your color put.

BONUS COLOR

Lipstick, even gloss, can be smudged or patted on your cheeks for a modern bit of blush. Here's a tip from the runway: clear gloss can look cool (for a moment) on both cheeks and as an eye gloss. Be careful not to make it too gooey.

glam lips

Try these looks for parties, dances, and other special occasions. Remember, if you go darker, brighter, or bolder with your lips, keep your eyes toned down and make sure your blush is gently applied. If you use pale lip colors, then you need darker eyes and should add a pop of pretty blush.

SHIMMER

Shimmery lipsticks or lip glosses make lips look lusciously full. A gloss with a hint of shimmer in your natural lip color is fine for the day. If you want to add some wattage when you go out, wear a product with shimmer that's a shade or two deeper or lighter than your ordinary gloss. Wear it alone for a simple, sheer look. Or experiment by layering it on top of different lipstick colors to see what you can come up with.

RED

Before you unleash that red lipstick from its tube or brandish the wand from a red gloss, the first thing you have to do is make sure your lips are ready for the red. Chapped lips look even worse when you apply red lipstick. So pamper that pucker by smoothing eye cream on lips; then use a toothbrush or a washcloth to gently exfoliate away any dry skin before you apply a really red lip.

For the reddest red, look for blue-red and orange-red shades of lipstick. This is the serious starlet red so make sure you have the attitude to go with it. Opt for a creamy, semi-matte formula rather than a totally matte lipstick. Typically, I'm not a fan of teens using a lip brush—it's just too high maintenance. But I'll make an exception when it comes to painting red lips. If you use a lip brush to apply the color, you'll be much more precise. And there's nothing worse than sloppy red lips. Apply lipstick on the center of the top lip and work outward to the corners. Brush the color on in thin layers, using short strokes. Repeat on the bottom lip. If you want to go even more intense, apply a second layer. Make sure you blot your lips with a tissue after the application to avoid getting any lipstick on your teeth.

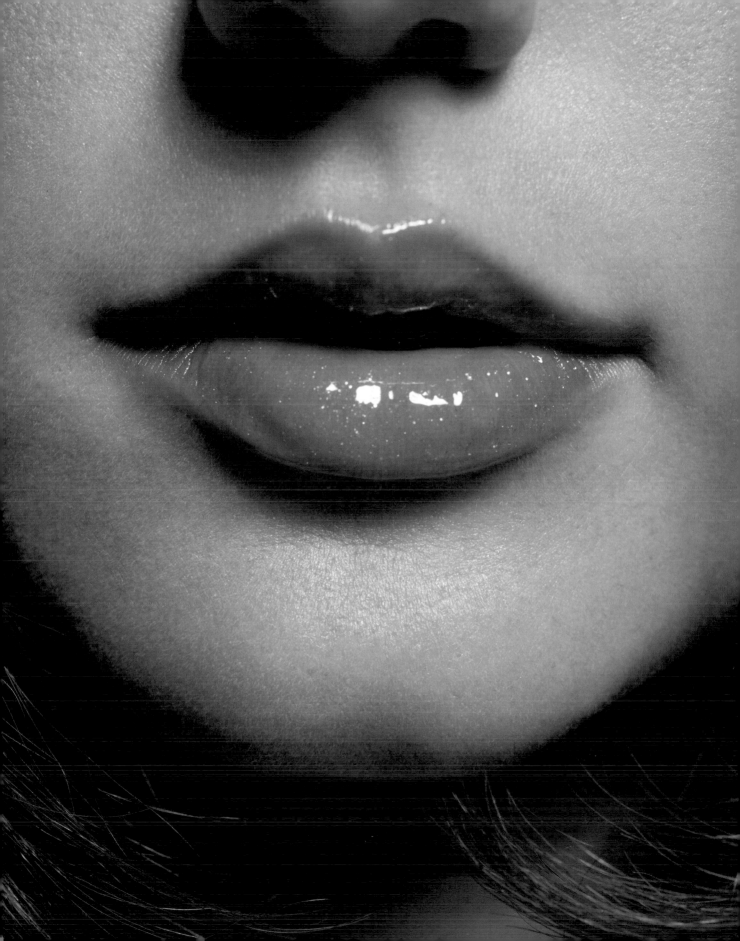

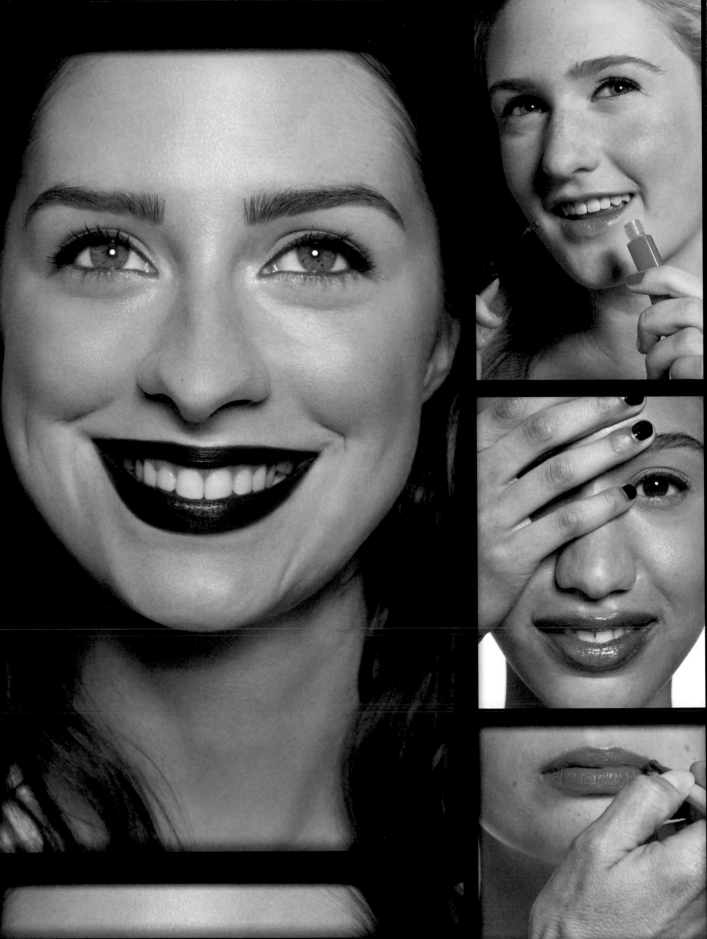

QUICK TIPS FOR BEAUTIFUL LIPS

TIP NUMBER 1:
SHEER GENIUS

SHEER COLORS, SUCH AS GLOSSES OR BALMS, ARE THE EASIEST WAY TO GET PRETTY LIPS.

TIP NUMBER 3:
THE LAYERED LOOK

LAYER GLOSS ON TOP OF LIPSTICK FOR A REALLY RICH POUT.

TIP NUMBER FIVE:
BALANCING ACT

Make sure your lips don't compete with your eye makeup. If you go for a strong eye, pair it with pale lips. Dark lips? Go easy on the eyes.

TIP NO. TWO:
SHINE ON

Change up your favorite lip gloss by adding a little sparkle.

TIP NUMBER 4:
LIGHTEN UP

IF YOU BUY A LIPSTICK THAT'S TOO DARK OR BRIGHT FOR YOUR TASTE, TURN IT INTO A STAIN. AFTER APPLYING THE LIPSTICK, BLOT MOST OF IT OFF FOR A SUBTLE AND LONG-LASTING COLOR.

TIP NUMBER SIX:
DOUBLE DUTY

Lipstick and gloss can be used as blush for a cool modern look (or in a pinch). But keep it light so you don't end up with sticky cheeks.

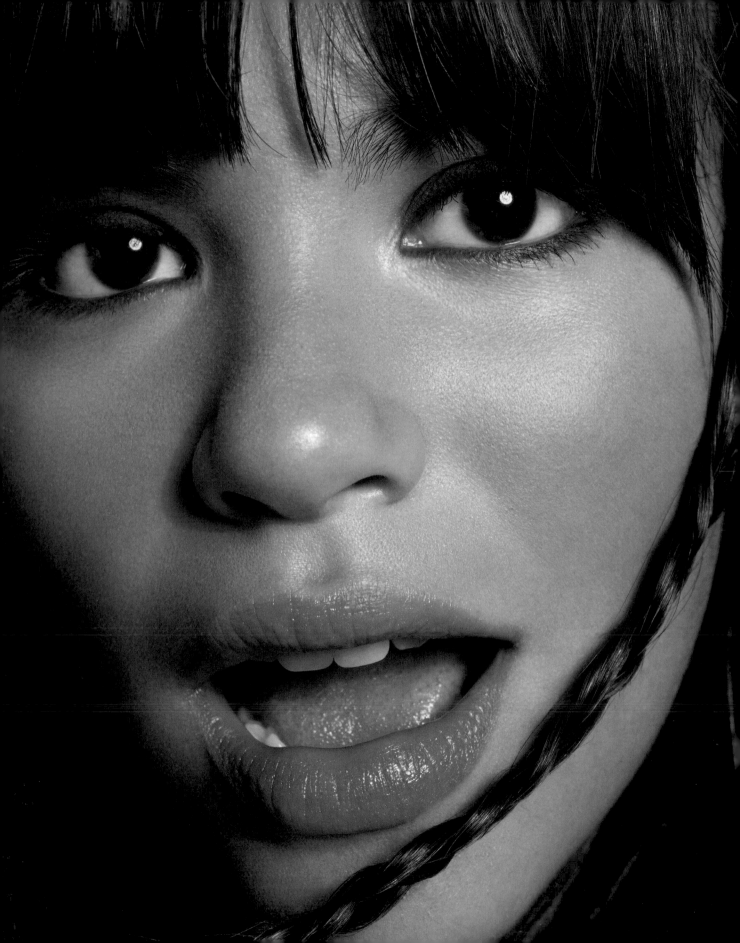

10

THE HAIR

The quest for perfect hair. I know it well. Growing up, we thought perfect hair meant long, stick-straight locks, parted down the middle. We used to iron our hair. We literally draped our hair over an ironing board, covered only by a towel, and took a hot clothing iron to it. Scary. Then there were the orange-juice cans that I used as rollers before I went to sleep. Not exactly comfortable, but all those sleepless nights seemed totally worth it to me at the time.

I know hair really defines you. When I've just had my hair blown out at the salon and it's totally shiny, that's the best. But I don't feel like I have to achieve that glossy perfection—the kind you see in magazines and on the red carpet—in my normal, everyday life. The secret to great-looking hair is embracing what you have naturally, keeping it super-healthy, and getting a great cut.

Accept and make the most of the hair you have. I couldn't be happier than when I'm able to help a girl, with amazing curly hair by wrestling the flat iron away and showing her the beauty of a tousled, sexy style. Going with your natural hair texture, and not against it, is how you get truly fabulous results.

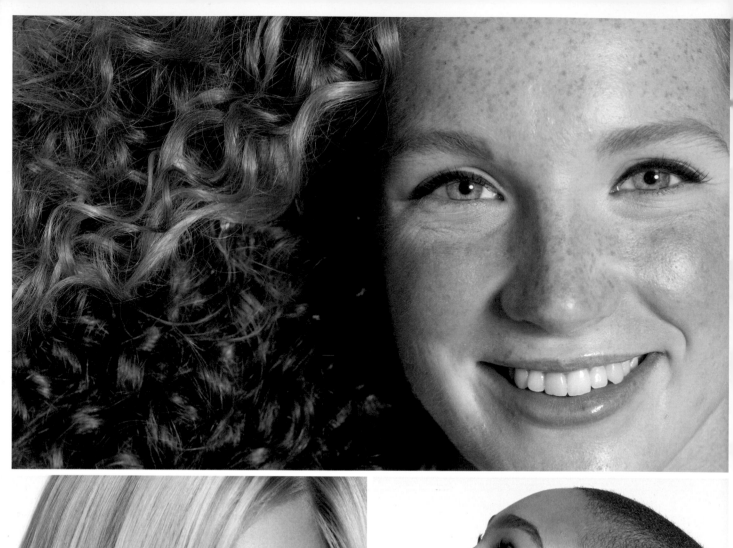

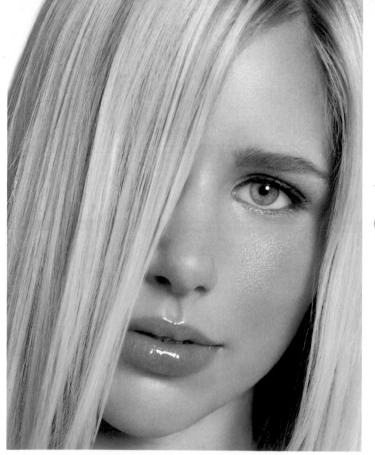

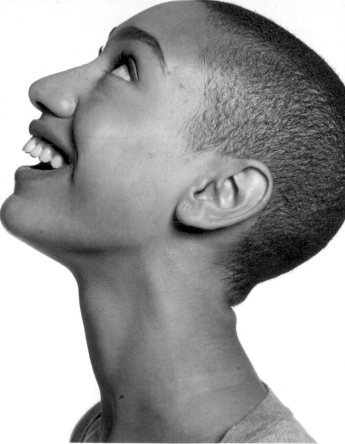

INTERVIEW: ERIC DOMINGUEZ
SECRETS FROM THE SALON

Eric Dominguez, who styled the hair on every page of this book (including my own), knows hair. We both believe that healthy, shiny hair is what is most beautiful. But what I love most about Eric is that he listens to what people want. So I always listen to his advice on hair, and so should you.

When it comes to hair, why does it seem like no one is happy with what they have on their head?

Hair is easy to blame. Hair is right there, looking terrible, when we wake up in the morning. It's an easy scapegoat. It's easy to feel bad about your hair when you look at magazines and celebrities, who have hairdressers at their disposal. Most people don't have the tools to get that kind of look. Even hairdressers ask one another to do their hair. It's just easier to have someone else do your hair.

What's a good way to be happy with the hair you have?

First, be honest about what you have. There is nothing wrong with wanting to change your hair. But look at the color, texture, and amount of hair you have, and try to find some attribute about it that you like. When people look at their faces to do their makeup, they try to highlight their best feature. Do the same when it comes to your hair, whether you have thick hair or an interesting color. Find one of those things and focus on that.

What do you think makes hair beautiful?

Healthy hair is always beautiful. It reflects the light beautifully. Anything that is good for skin is good for hair—a good diet, a lot of water, exercise. Also minimal abuse is important. That means limiting sun exposure, friction from brushing, flat irons, or hair dryers. When it comes to those last two tools, ask your hairdresser about what temperature settings to use. If you have fine hair, you can't crank the heat up.

How does hair complement style? What does it show about a person?

It is an instant way of expressing ourselves. When a girl has a passion about waking up in the morning and using her hair as a tool for expression, like an artist, then I say go for it. I think girls with pink or green hair are gorgeous because they become a living coloring book. But I also think it's beautiful to see a young jock—who grows her hair long and her hair is healthy because she is healthy—wearing her hair in a ponytail like a lovely piece of fabric flowing down her back. Get to know what style you want and don't let anyone alter that.

What's the best way to find your own hairstyle?

The secret is knowing what you are willing to put into your hair. There are women who can color their own hair or work an iron like nobody's business. If you are not that proficient, or not interested in spending a half an hour every morning doing your hair, get a simple haircut that fits your style.

How can girls find a good hairstylist?

Here's one of my favorite ways to find a hairdresser that I tell all my clients moving to a new city where I don't know any salons. Go to the nicest department store you can find and head to the makeup department. Look for one of the girls behind the counter whose hair is in great shape and who has a great cut. Then ask who cuts her hair. These women are in the public eye all day long, and they're discerning. In most cases, they are also pretty demanding. You will find a hairdresser who can listen and communicate. And that's what you want—a hairdresser who can bring out what you want when you wake up and look in the mirror.

Any tips on how to get the haircut you want once you walk into the salon?

There's nothing wrong with bringing pictures from magazines. But you want to find someone whose hair is the same texture and density as yours. If you have thick hair and you walk in with a picture of fine, windblown hair, that's never going to happen.

Isn't a picture of a celebrity or fashion model an unrealistic example?

I always suggest that people cut the person's face and body out of the picture and just have the hair. Or if you aren't that crafty, stick a piece of paper over the face. You don't want the hairdresser thinking you want to look like the model or actress. You want them to focus in on the hair. They will see the frame you are trying to create and not the latest celebrity. Just as you are focusing in on the hair, they will then focus in on the hair and remove any preconceived ideas.

What can a girl do if she gets a really, really bad haircut?

Use it as an opportunity to try something you might never do otherwise. If you always wear your hair long and get a crummy medium-length haircut, find a hairdresser through someone who always has a great haircut and say, "I am hating this so much; I can't hate anything more." Then go for it. Try a short cut or layers. Sometimes growing out a bad cut back to the way your hair was before is not the best thing to do. Follow that initial desire to change by changing again.

What's your advice for girls with stick-straight hair?

I love really short, French-schoolboy haircuts that you see in fashion magazines. They are simple. You just remove hair being an issue. If someone wants to wear her hair longer, a beautiful crisp blunt haircut is always classic. It always looks clean and healthy. If your hair is also really thick, like Asian hair, find a hairstylist who is proficient with a straight razor. With a straight-razor cut, you get a lot of movement and softness. You wind up having very little maintenance. You wake up with style.

How about curly or wavy hair?

If you don't want to get into a production every morning, always wear it curly. Don't blow it out once a week. You will end up disturbing the curl. Only comb or brush your hair once a week in the shower. Use your fingers or a wide-tooth comb to get the snags out. Brushing stretches the curl, which makes it look frizzy. If you can go one or two days without shampooing it, just wet your hair. This will bring the natural oils down throughout the hair shaft, making it look shiny. The curls will also be more defined and less frizzy. You can use conditioner, which will remove the perspiration and dust from hair while still maintaining the curl.

What are some easy ways to change up anyone's hair?

Ponytails are great. If you wear one high or low, it immediately changes what you see, even from the front. Hair accessories are another way to get creative. I had a girl who brought in an antique belt buckle to put into her hair for an event. Experiment by attaching objects found at flea markets to bobby pins and fabric-covered rubber bands. You won't find the same stuff on other people's heads.

Is it possible to get glam hair that's not too fussy?

Divide and conquer. If you wanted to put your hair up, divide the hair from ear to ear. Take the front half and get it out of the way and ignore it. Take the hair behind the ears and put it a ponytail or pin it in a knot shape. Once that's out of the way, take the front hair and gently pull sections back with combs or bobby pins. The bottom section is your foundation. And there are no rules for the front section, so have fun. Girls with curly hair have it the easiest. You can just start pinning it up. Get strong clips and let it be messy and tumbling down.

Why should girls love their own hair?

I'm Latin American, and there are all different types of hair in my family. I have a sister with the hair texture of an African American. Growing up, she would chemically straighten her hair and wasn't allowed to go in the pool if we had something important to do the next day. That really limited her. It is important to embrace what you have. It doesn't mean you can't get your hair done differently. There's nothing wrong with that. But if you can accept that "I'm still beautiful with what grows out of my head naturally," you'll gain a lot of freedom.

DON'T OVERTHINK OR OVERWORK YOUR HAIR.

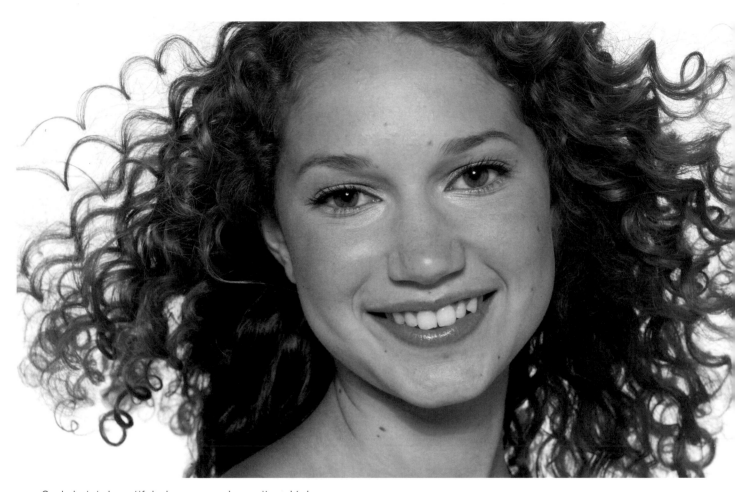

Curly hair is beautiful when you embrace it and take good care of it. Never brush curly hair when it's dry. Detangle curls when hair is wet and has conditioner in it. For amazing curls like these, wrap sections around your finger while the hair is still wet to define the curl. Then let it air-dry so you don't disturb the natural curl.

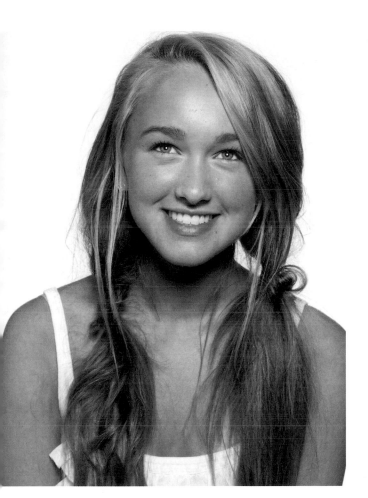

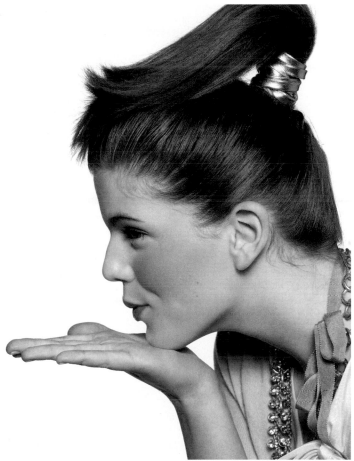

Pigtails can be cool and modern. Keep the pigtails loose so there's volume toward the face, and tie the fasteners at your shoulders. If you want to get advanced, wrap a section of hair around the rubber band to make it part of the accessory. Don't sweat fly-aways. They add to the soft and casual look.

Hair accessories can be simple, elegant, and fun. Here two gold headbands are wrapped around and turned into a ponytail holder that adds drama. Be creative with your accessories. Try ties, brooches, belts, anything you like.

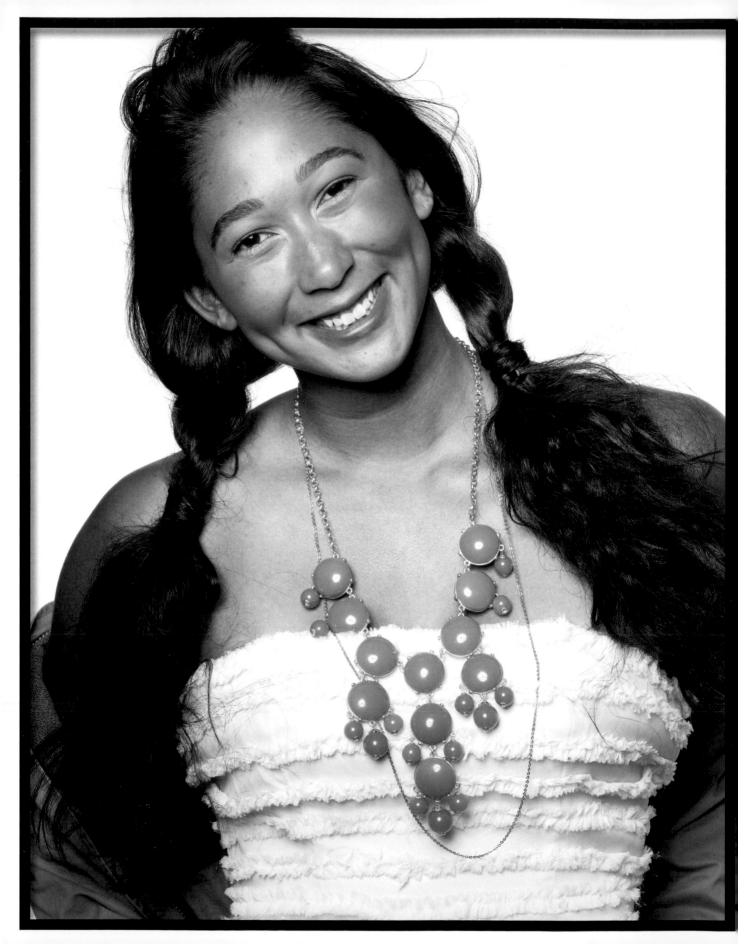

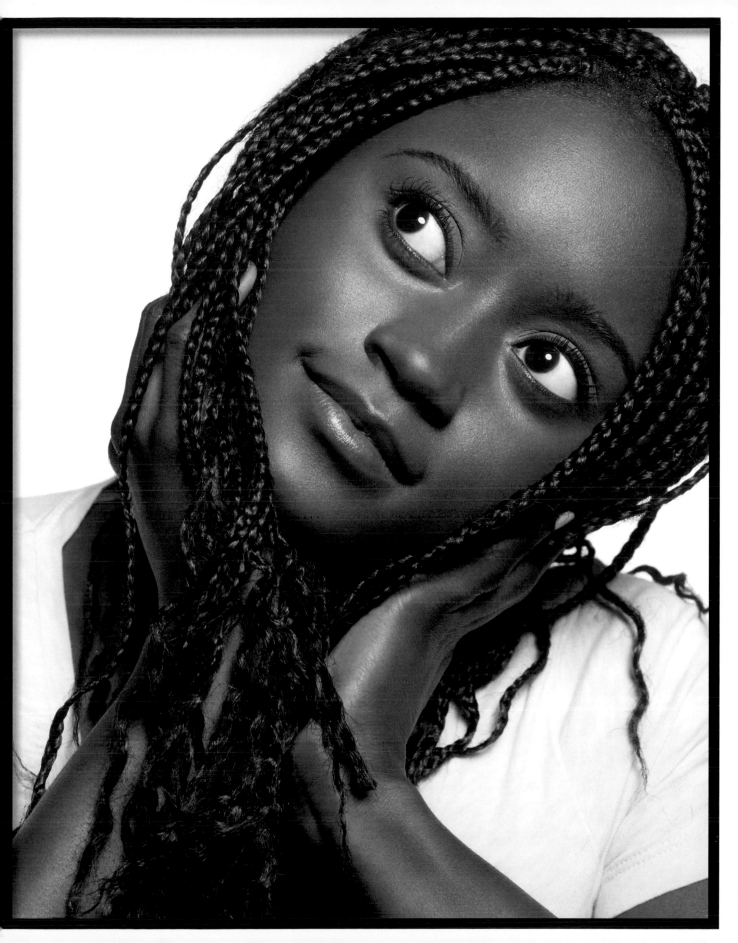

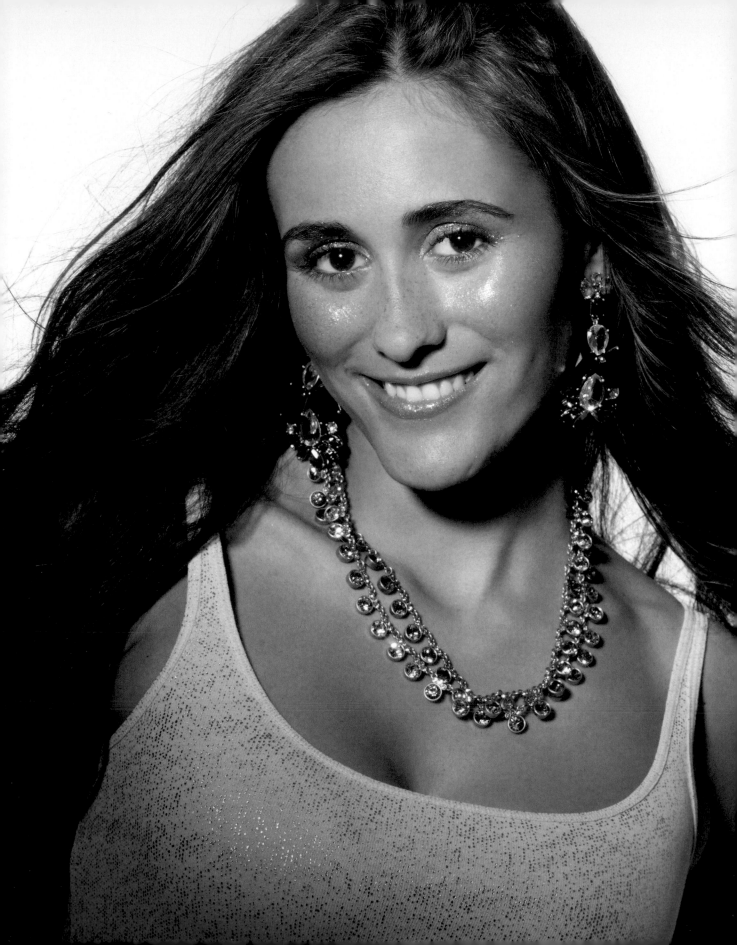

BOBBI + ERIC'S QUICK TIPS FOR TERRIFIC HAIR

TIP NUMBER 1:

HEALTHY IS BEAUTIFUL

SHINY, GLOSSY, GLORIOUS—ANYTHING THAT IS GOOD FOR YOUR BODY IS GOOD FOR YOUR HAIR. AND THAT'S GOOD FOR YOUR LOOK.

TIP NO. TWO:

DON'T WASH YOUR HAIR EVERY DAY

There's no need to unless you work in construction. You wake up every morning and rinse it with warm water and conditioner, which will remove dust and perspiration. At most, wash every other day.

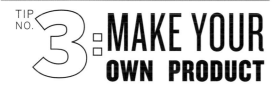

TIP NO. 3: MAKE YOUR OWN PRODUCT

Mixing a couple of products together in your hand is a really great way to create something that works for your individual hair texture. Try combining a little mousse with some gel, or pomade and hair cream. Experiment to find out what gives your hair that perfect look. Good old-fashioned moisturizer is a great way to tame fly-aways.

TIP NUMBER 4: THE MOST IMPORTANT HAIR ACCESSORY

in the universe is a cloth-covered rubber band. It's cool to have messy hair in a bun or ponytail.

TIP NO. 5: DON'T BURN OUT

Give your flat iron a rest. Hair is like fabric, which gets ruined if you iron it every day. Take a break and wear it back for a couple of days. Buy really good conditioners. Only use straightening irons with a thermostat, and never let it go over 180 or 200 degrees, or you will singe your hair.

TIP NUMBER SIX: WORD OF MOUTH

IS THE BEST WAY TO FIND A GREAT HAIRDRESSER. TALK TO PEOPLE WHO HAVE THE SAME KIND OF HAIR YOU HAVE OR A GREAT CUT.

TIP NUMBER SEVEN:

When you don't spend too much time fussing with and thinking about your hair, that's when you find beauty. Hairdressers go to where young people hang out to find the girl who, having left dance class, has her hair falling out of the bun. Or there's the girl who is growing out her bangs and wearing it messy in a clip. Those are the hairstyles that inspire us.

TIP NUMBER EIGHT: THERE IS ALWAYS GOING TO BE SOMEONE WHO LIKES YOUR HAIR THE OTHER WAY

YOU NEED TO BE ABLE TO LOOK IN THE MIRROR AND SAY, "I LOVE THE WAY I LOOK."

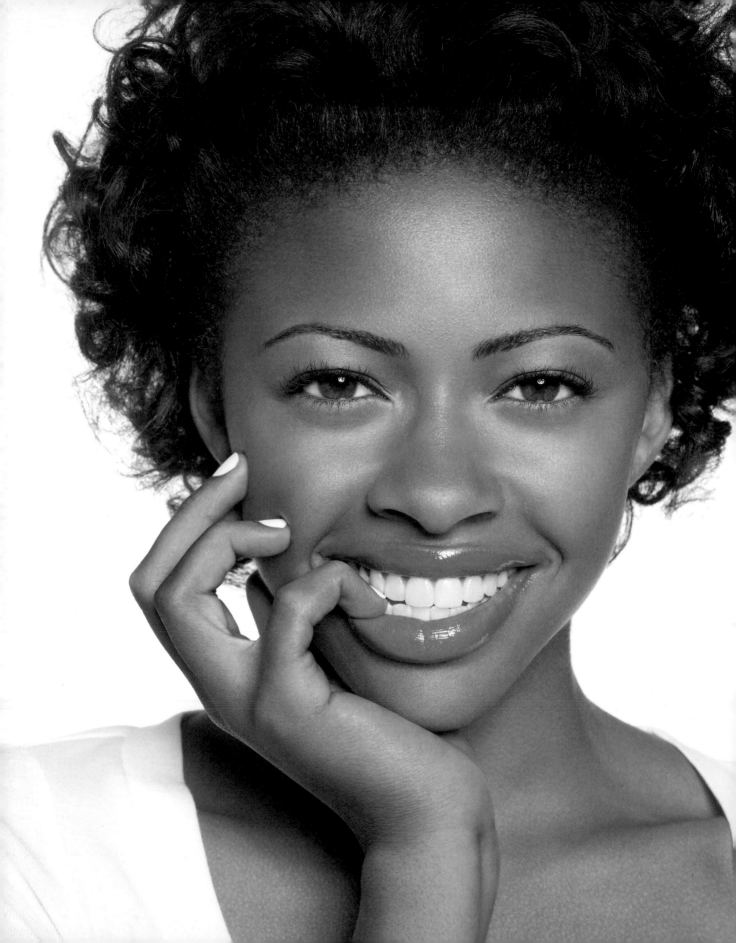

11

MAKEOVERS

Makeover is such a misleading word. Most of the time what makes someone look better is actually only a few tweaks, like using concealer or lining the eyes. *Makeover* implies starting over. Okay, sometimes there are a *lot* of tweaks in making an improvement to a person's looks. But because I truly believe that all girls are beautiful, all it really takes is knowledge, skill, and the right colors to make us look even better. It's pretty simple. Check out these before and afters.

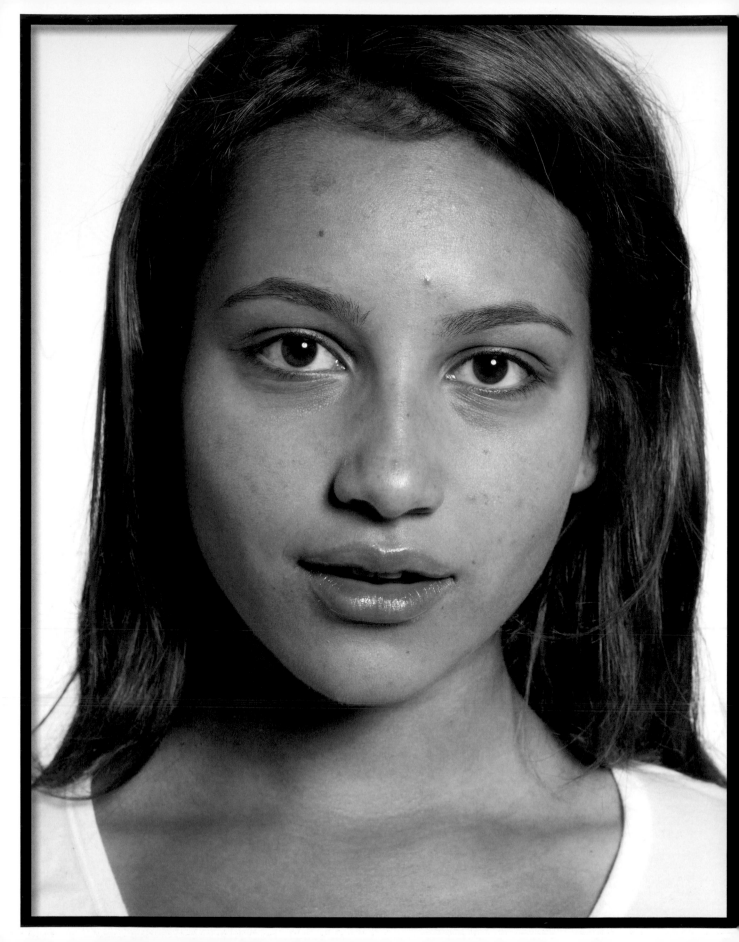

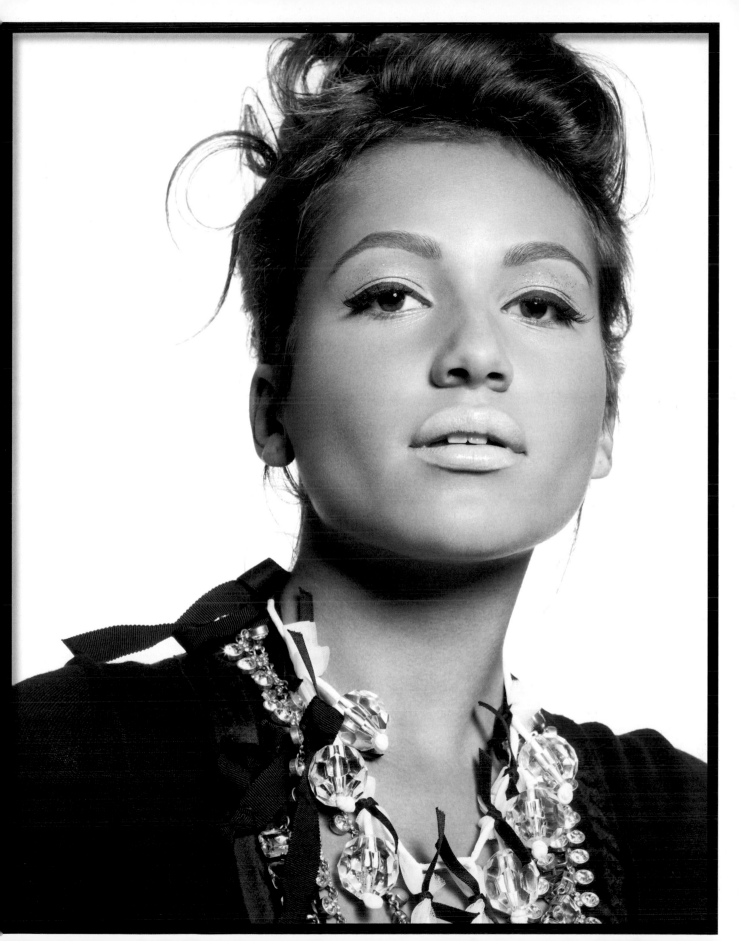

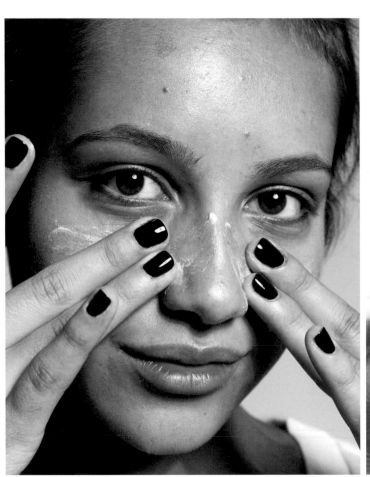

Always start with a light moisturizer.

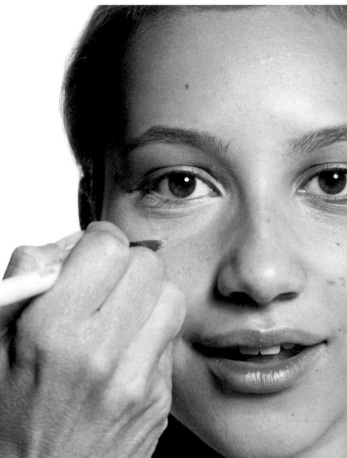

I lightened up the area under Nadia's eye with concealer, which made a big difference.

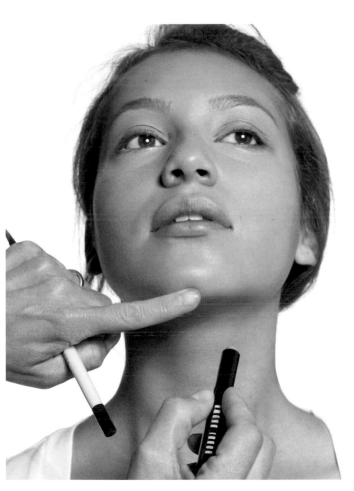

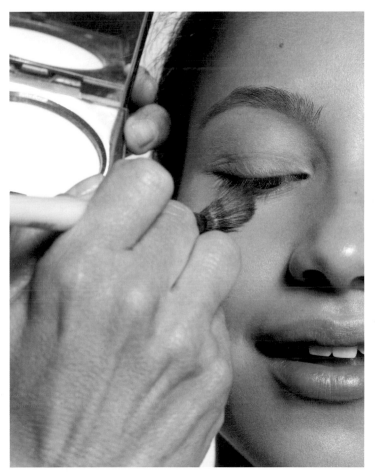

I applied foundation all over her face to even out her olive skin tone. Then I used a touch-up stick on any stubborn spots.

I applied yellow powder over the concealer, around Nadia's nose, and in her T-zone to get rid of any shine and help the makeup last.

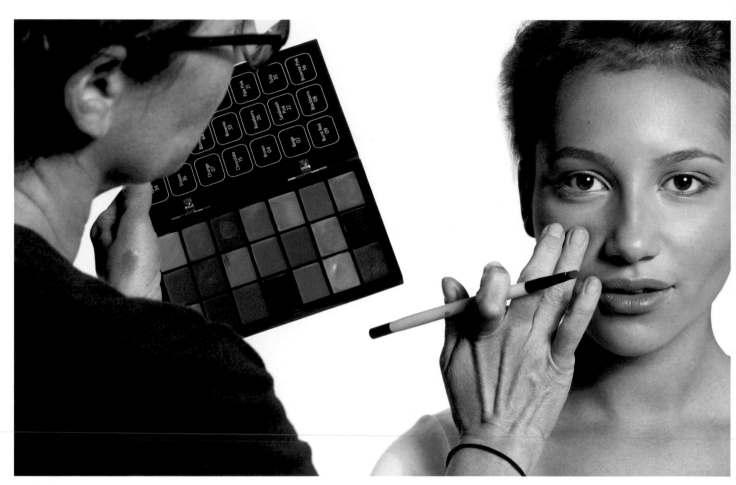

I used a pinkish cream blush on her cheeks. She had
naturally pinkish lips, so I applied a warm beige lipstick to
tone down the color because I wanted to play up her eyes.

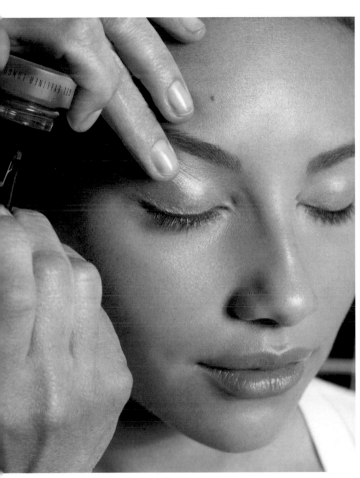

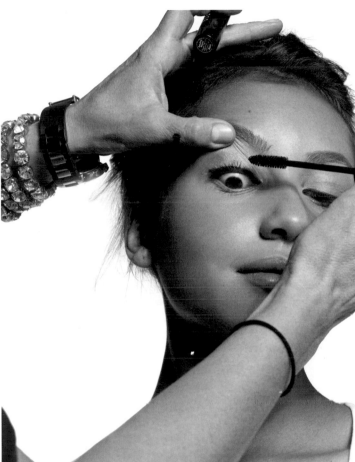

I filled in Nadia's brow and applied a cream shimmer shadow on her lids. The best way to put on cream eye shadow is with a synthetic brush or a fingertip, which gives a denser application. I followed that up by lining her eyes in dark brown.

A couple of coats of black mascara completes the look.

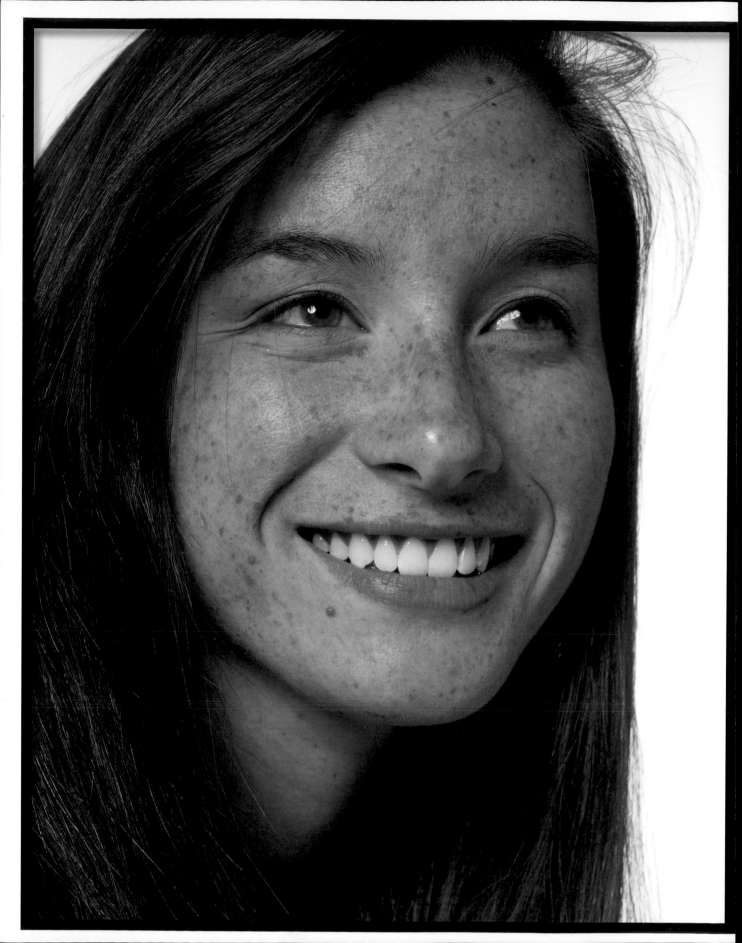

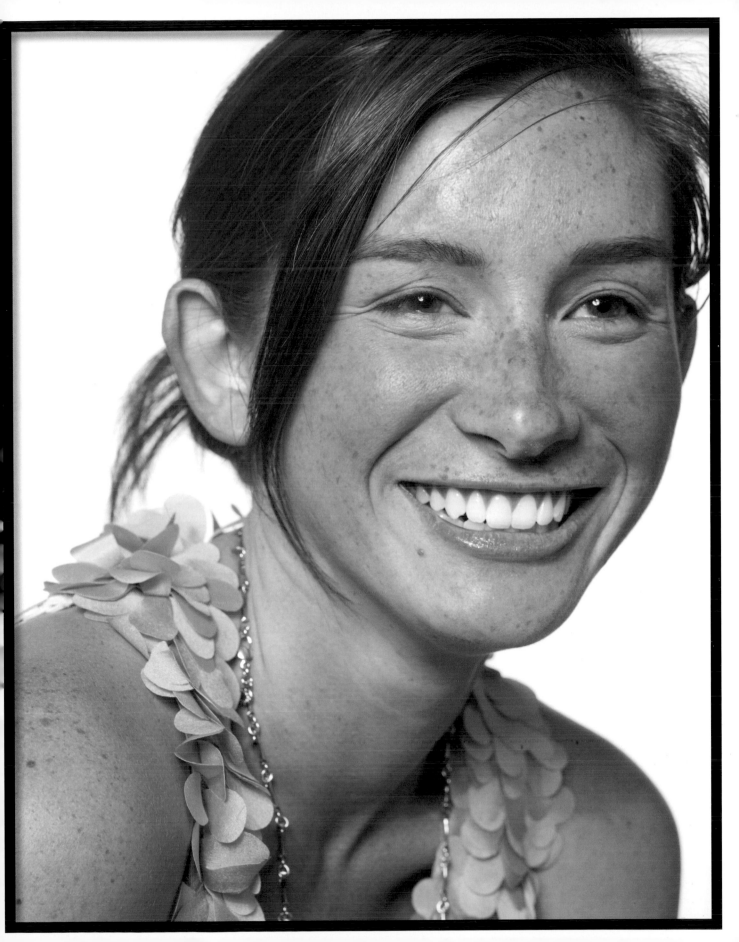

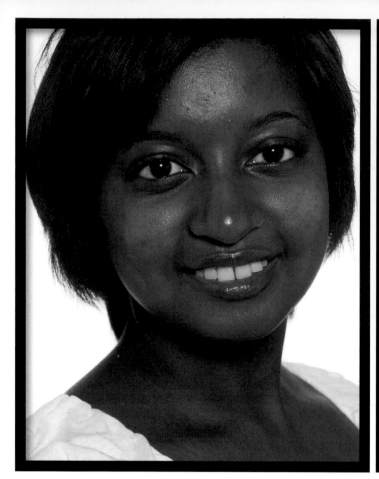

BEFORE:

Justine has an open face that exudes warmth.

AFTER:

I brightened under her eyes with a corrector and concealer. Then I applied foundation to even out her skin naturally. Her eyes look so pretty with a couple of shadow tones blended together and neat black liner. I used a cinnamon blush on her cheeks and a honey lipstick on her lips.

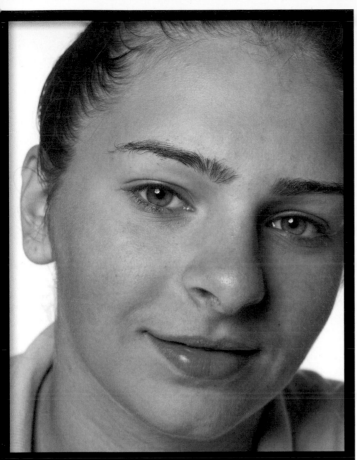 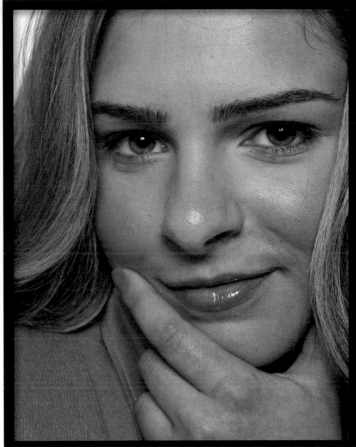

BEFORE:

Hannah has amazing skin that tans easily.

AFTER:

I kept the glow going by adding a peachy blush to her cheeks. For a little extra polish, we shaped, trimmed, and brushed up her eyebrows. Nail polish is a great way to add bold color. Hannah picked a bright orange, which worked well with her clothes.

NICOLE

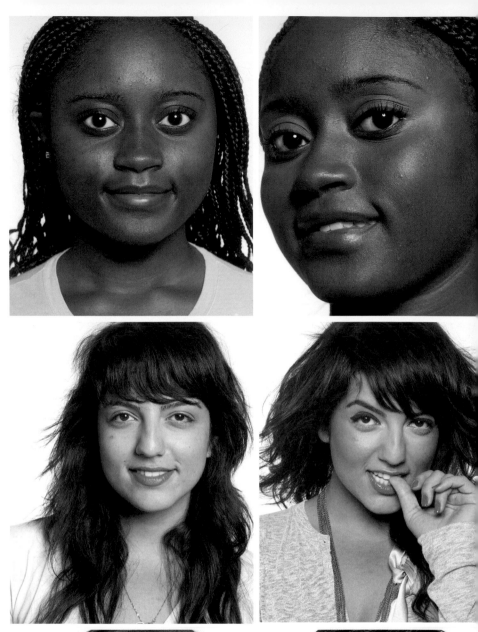

SUNNY

ANNA

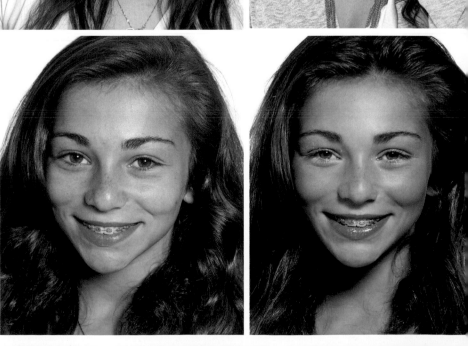

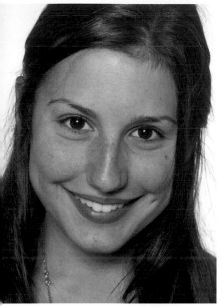
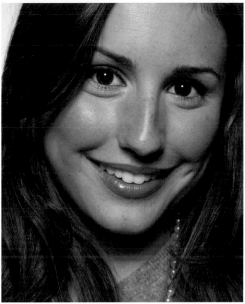

MADDIE

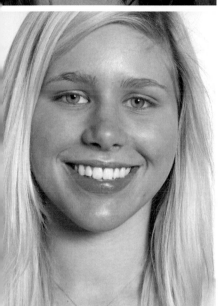
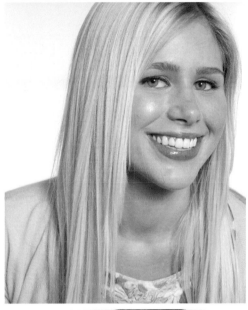

ELIZABETH

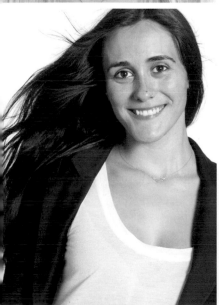
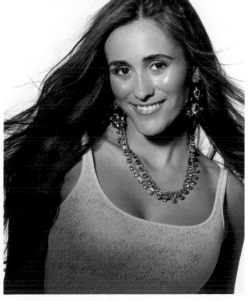

DANIELLA

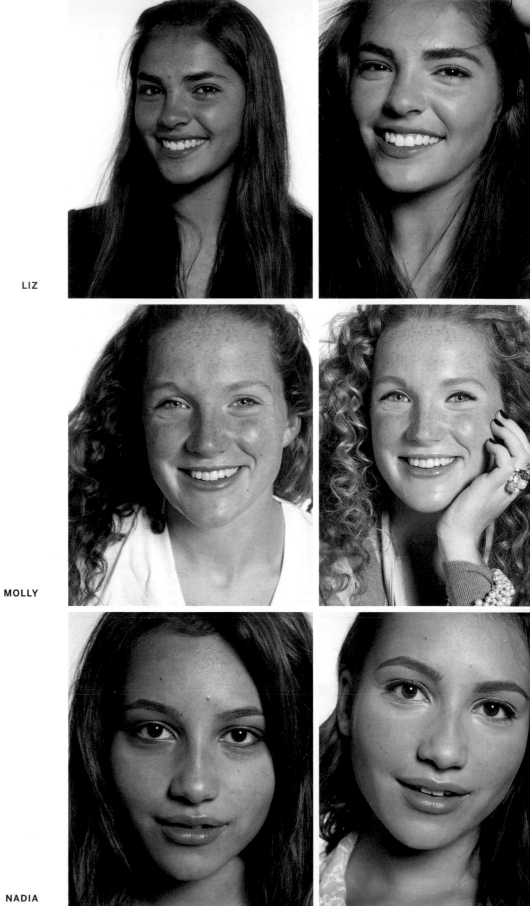

LIZ

MOLLY

NADIA

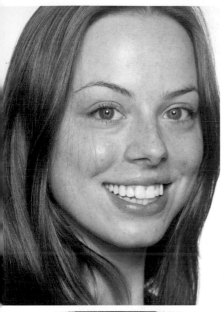
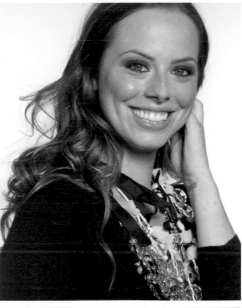

EMILY

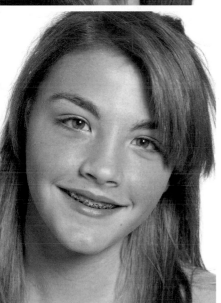
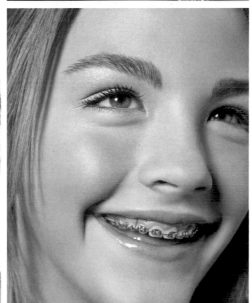

DANI

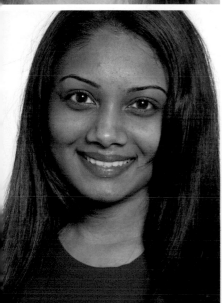
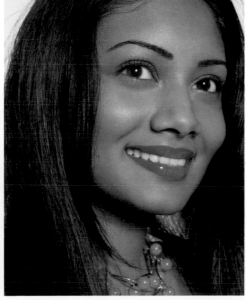

MELISSA

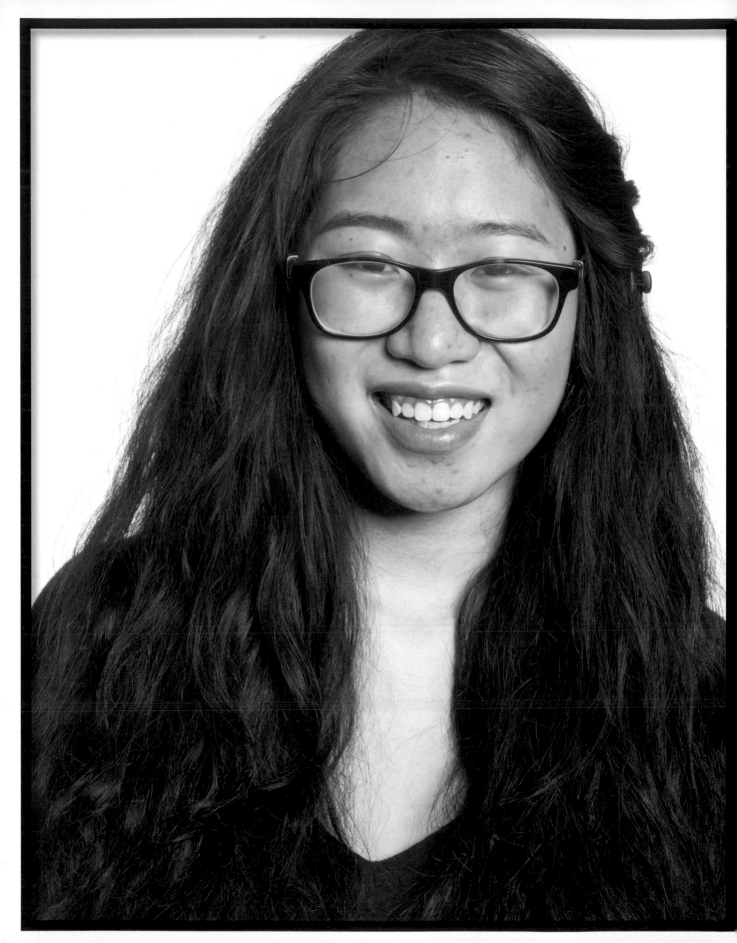

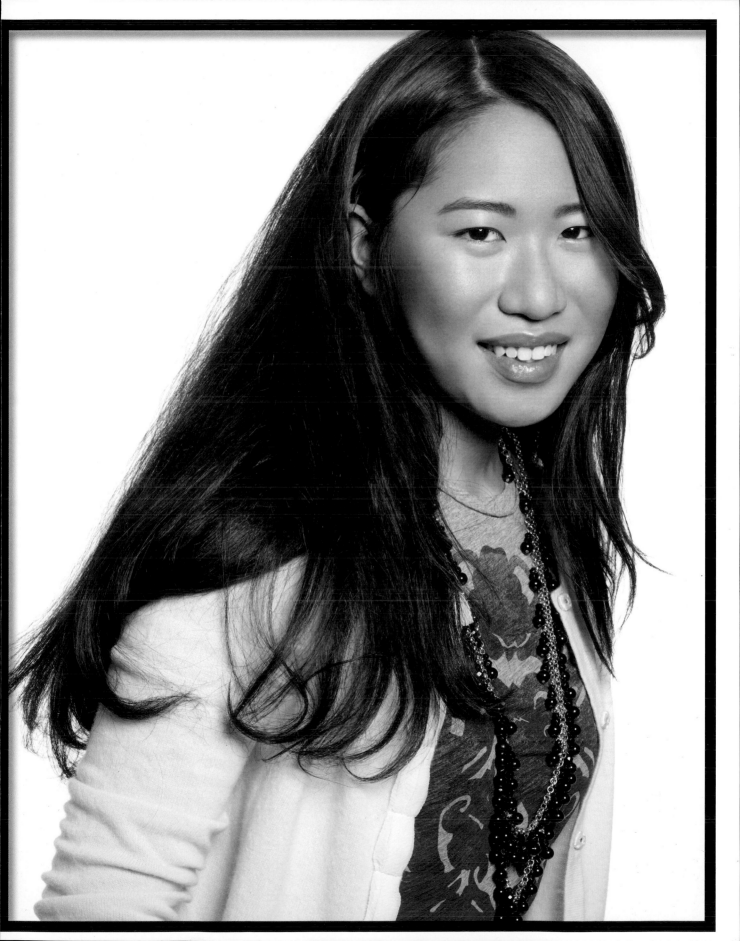

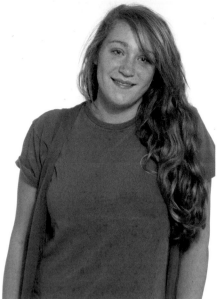

BEFORE:

Nolan is a natural beauty, but she didn't realize how pretty she is.

AFTER:

By evening out her skin and giving her a soft, smoky eye, her beauty came shining through. Her strong personality and understated look complement each other perfectly.

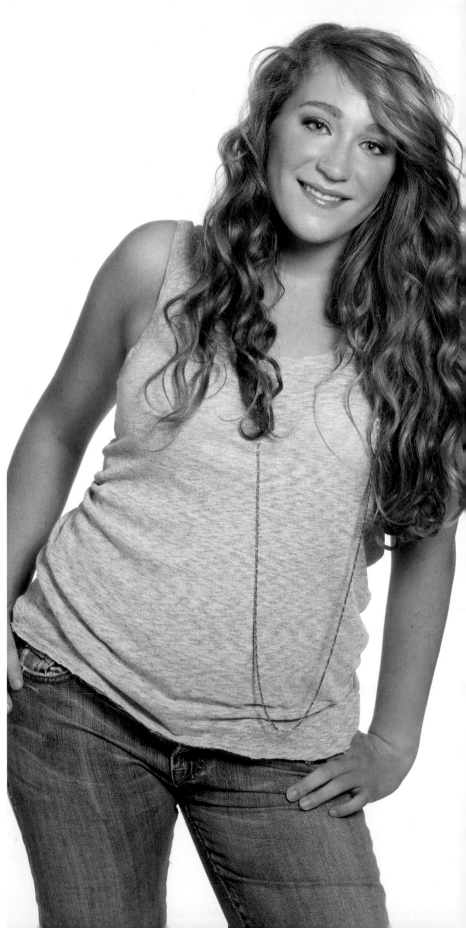

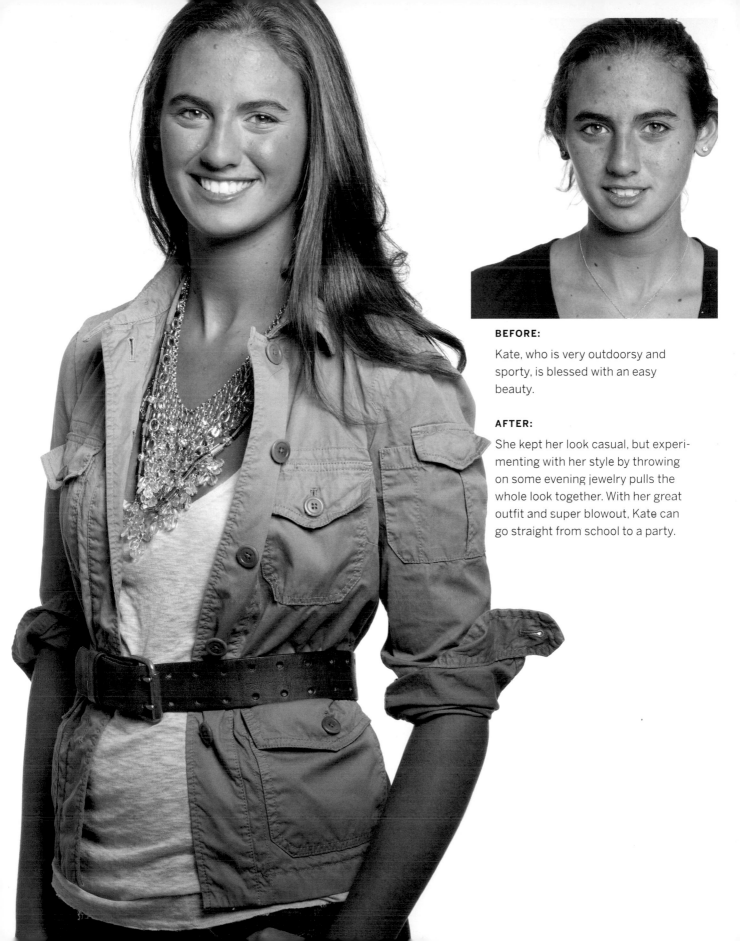

BEFORE:

Kate, who is very outdoorsy and sporty, is blessed with an easy beauty.

AFTER:

She kept her look casual, but experimenting with her style by throwing on some evening jewelry pulls the whole look together. With her great outfit and super blowout, Kate can go straight from school to a party.

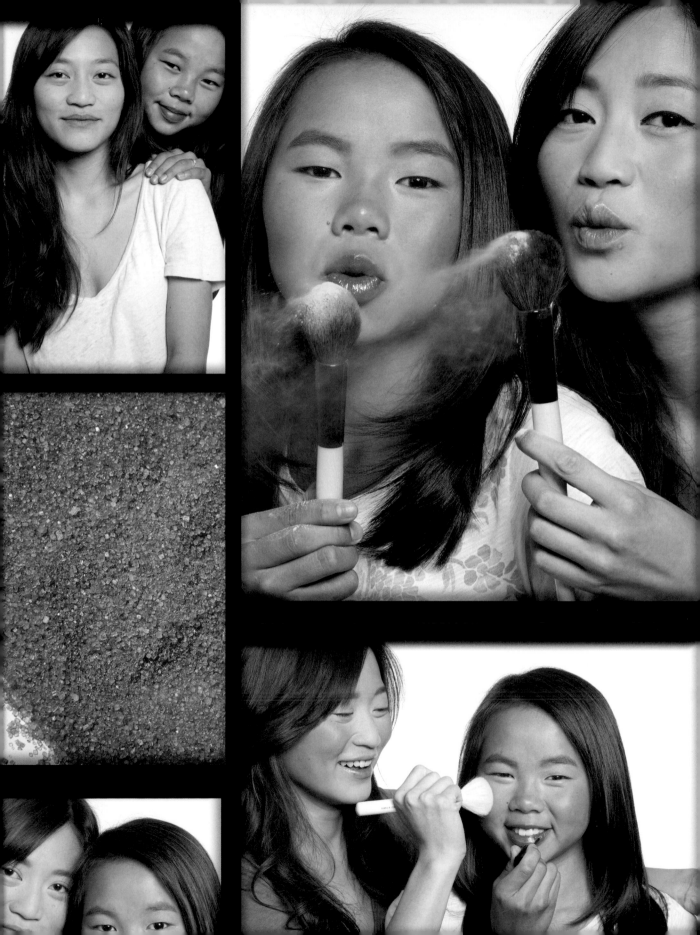

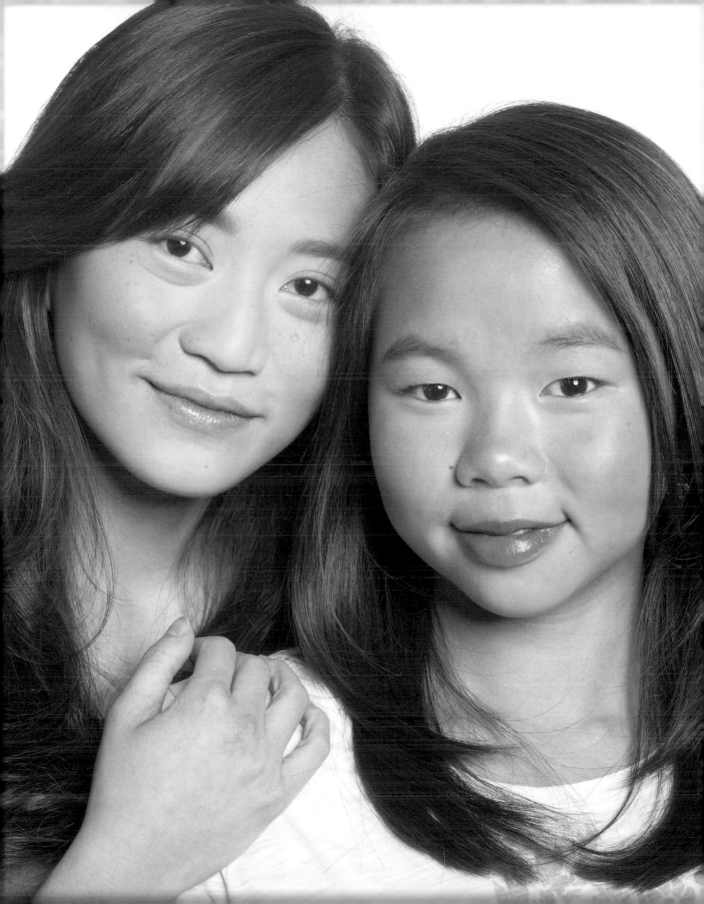

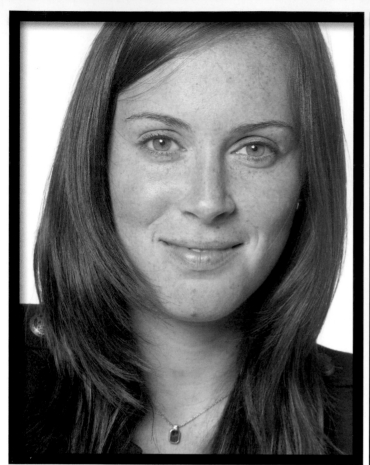

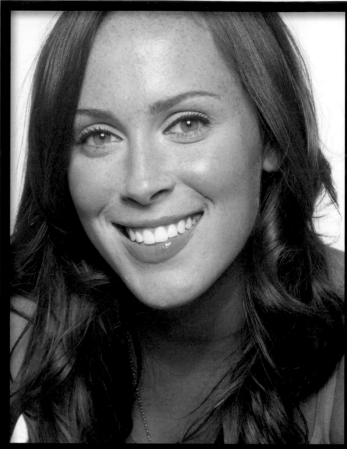

BEFORE:

Cierra looks so good without makeup. She has tons of freckles, which I love.

AFTER:

I left her eyes light with a strong liner and softly filled in her brows. With tinted moisturizer and shine on her cheeks and lips, she looks polished and beautiful.

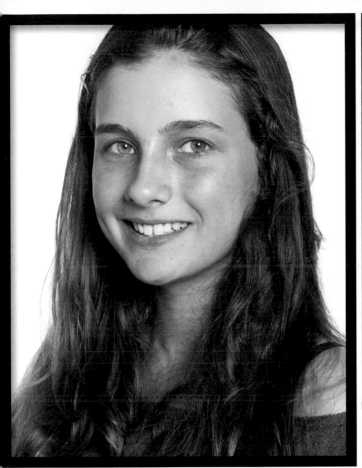 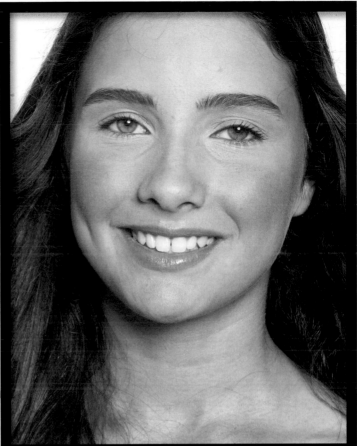

BEFORE:

Sima looks like a very young Brooke Shields. She has beautiful eyebrows.

AFTER:

I made her brows even stronger by filling them in, which framed her eyes. The rest of her makeup is nude to add to the effect.

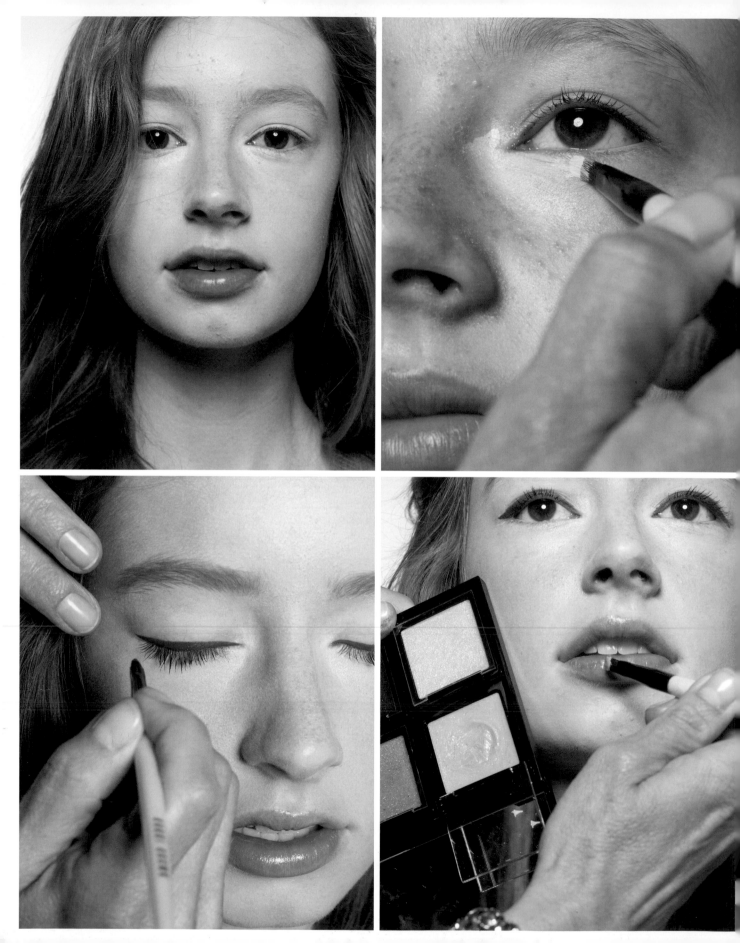

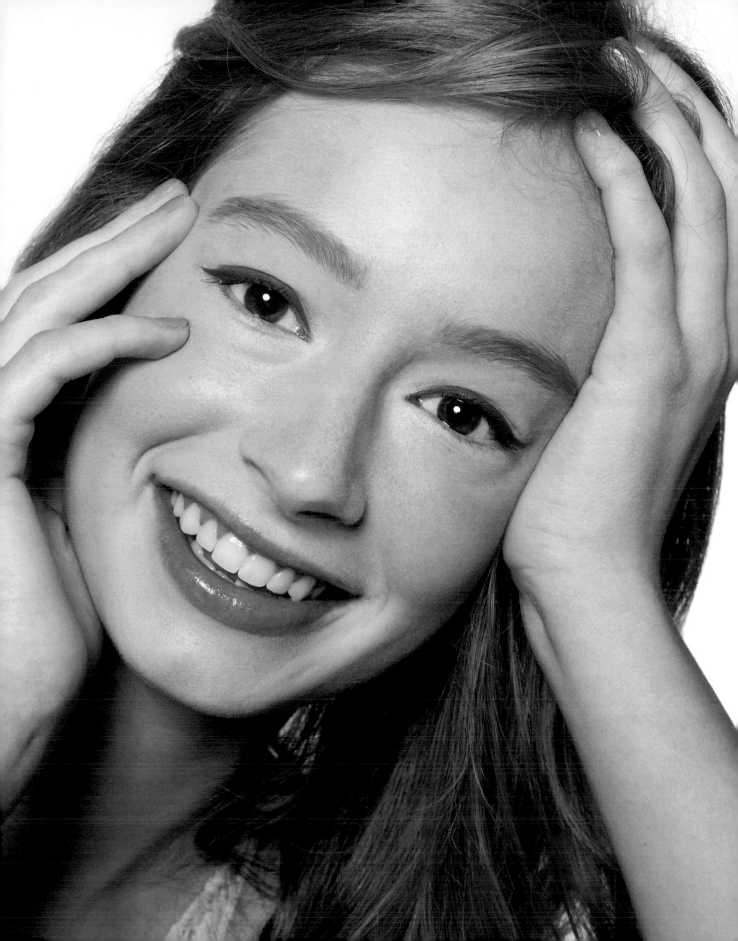

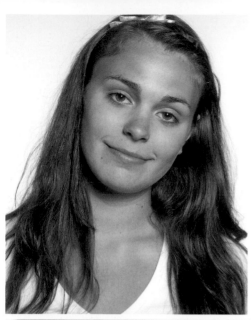

BEFORE:

Christina has amazing brown eyes that match her amazing spirit. (For more on Christina's charity, Dresses with Dignity, see page 222).

AFTER:

I used a bone eye shadow on her lower lids with peach shadow just above to complement her natural coloring. I followed that with mahogany brown eyeliner and mascara on her top lashes only.

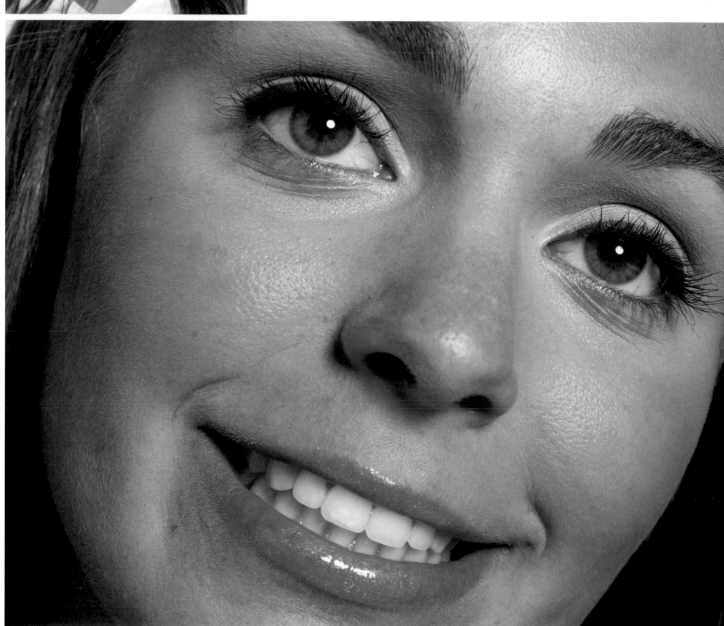

BEFORE:

The bright, clear blue of Gabby's eyes are breathtaking.

AFTER:

With her ringlets and perfect skin, Gabby reminded me of a fairy princess. So I used sheer tinted moisturizer to even out her complexion and focused on bringing out her natural pink cheeks. Then I went to town with sparkle—on her eyes, cheeks, and even her hair.

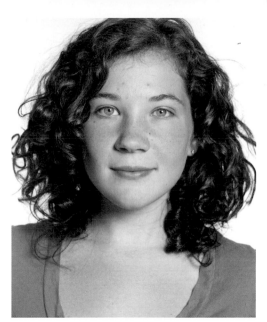

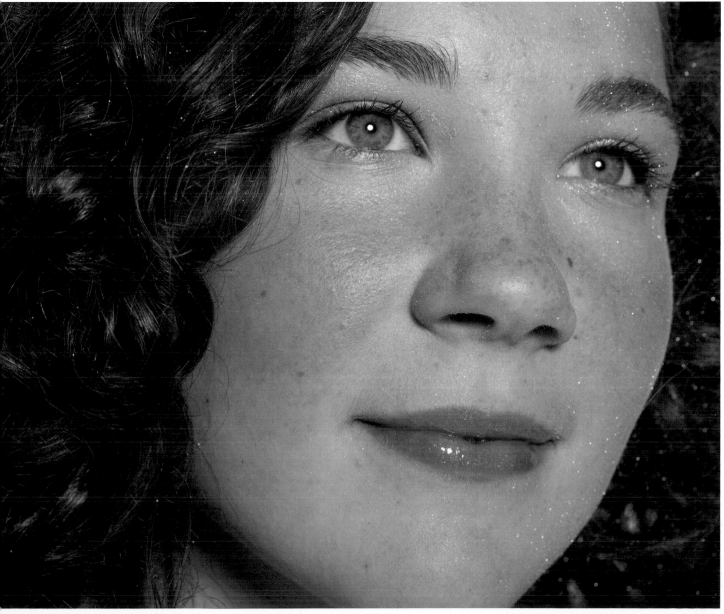

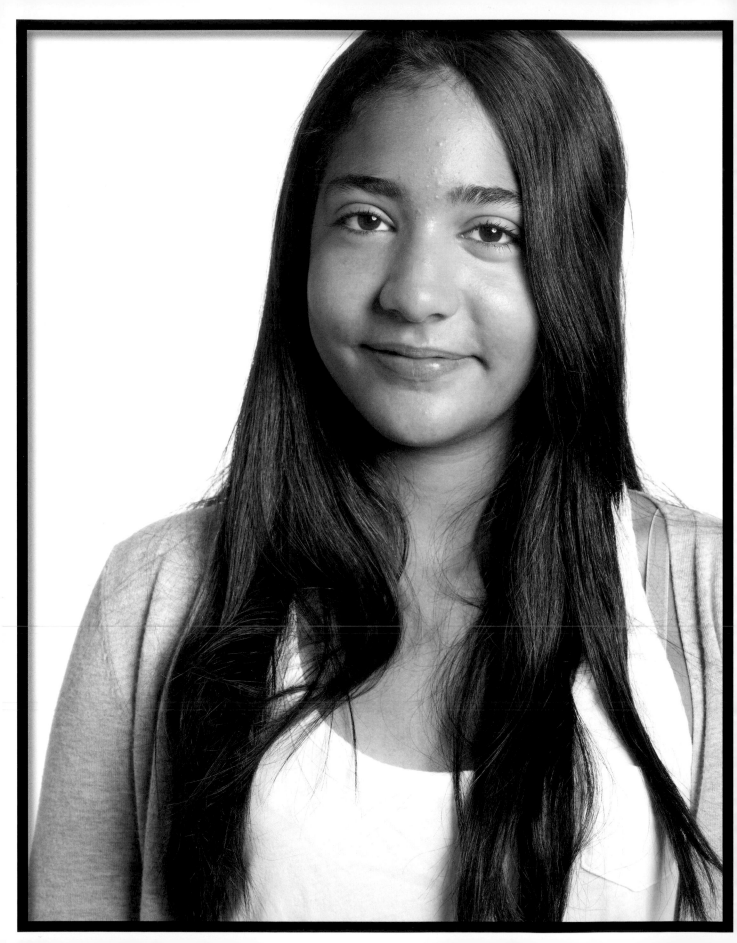

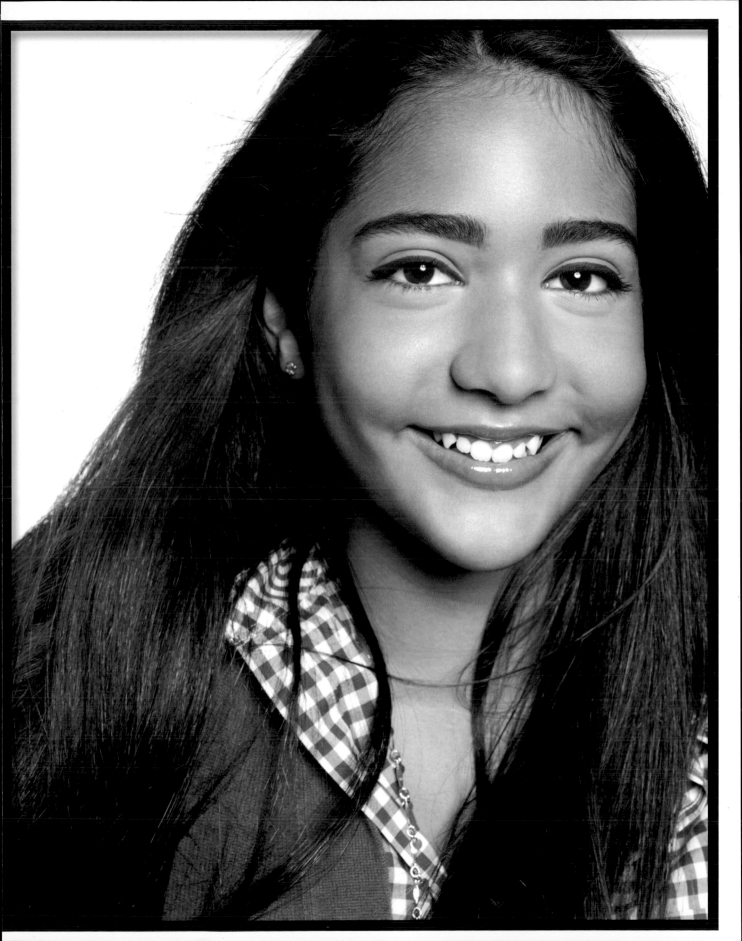

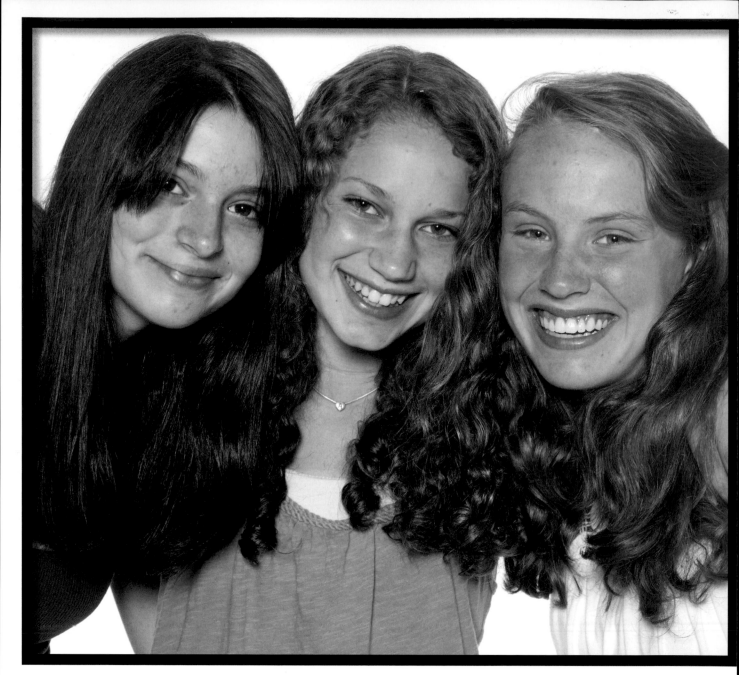

BEFORE:

Aurora, Amelia, and Lena are three fresh-faced beauties
with super-sweet smiles.

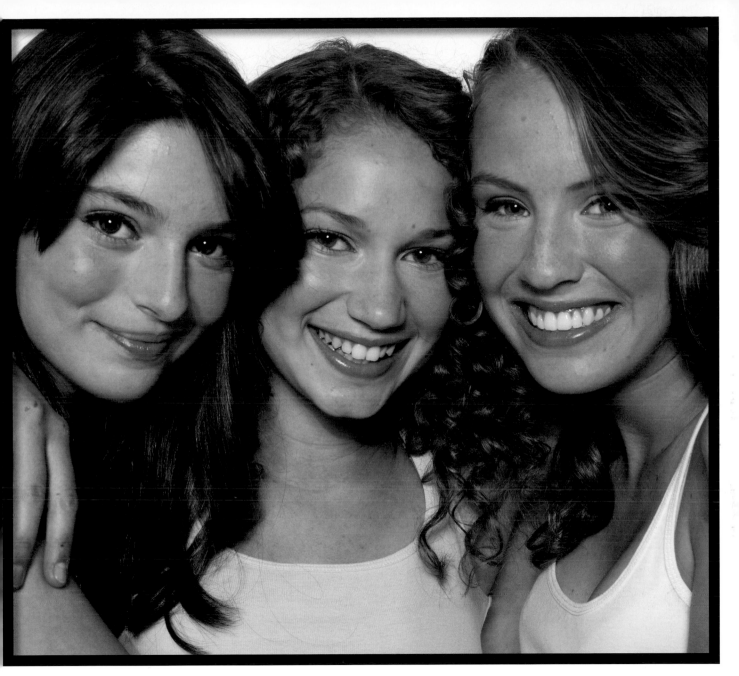

AFTER:

I matched their natural beauty with natural-looking and minimal makeup that simply lets these friends shine.

BEFORE:

Keira's thick hair frames her perfectly shaped face. And that skin!

AFTER:

I kept her face really fresh by applying a tinted moisturizer all over. I didn't use any liner, just a bunch of coats of mascara that gave her eyes plenty of definition. It looks really natural and shows how just evening out the skin and adding mascara make a big difference.

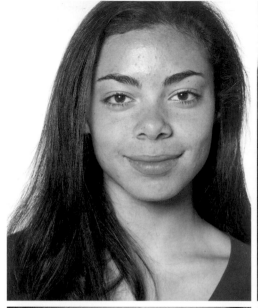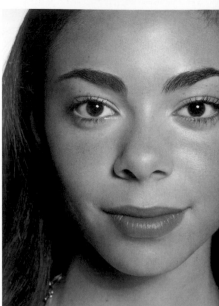

BEFORE:

Amanda is fortunate to have an amazing smile. I absolutely love her dimples.

AFTER:

Her eyes are really soulful and deep set, so I lined only the top to make them stand out.

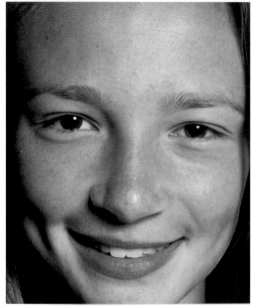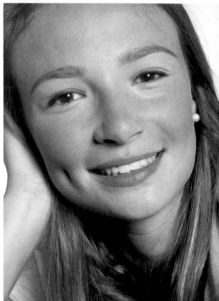

BEFORE:

Jillian's beauty mark is her signature, a punctuation on her amazing skin.

AFTER:

Because she has flawless skin, no foundation was needed. I just brushed up her gorgeous thick eyebrows, added mascara, blush, and some lipgloss, and the look was complete.

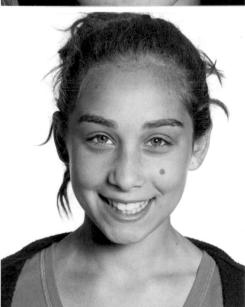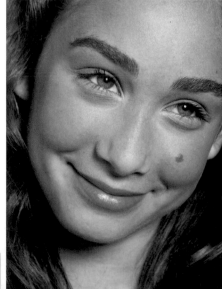

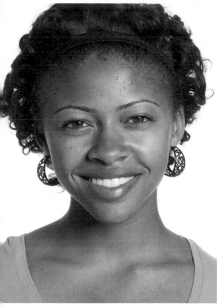
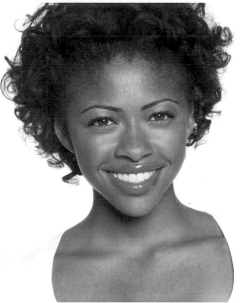

BEFORE:

Danielle has a great smile, beautiful teeth, and flawless skin.

AFTER:

A natural foundation that evened out her coloring allowed her eyes to pop. I kept everything true to her skin color, lined her upper lids, and smudged a little eye shadow on the lower lashes. Her hair made a big difference. Loosened up, it's softer, modern, and frames her face nicely.

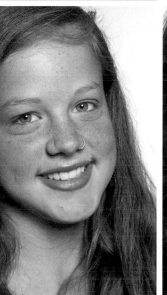
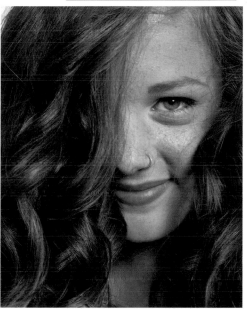

BEFORE:

Ana has the freckled, outdoorsy look, so I was surprised by the edgy nose ring.

AFTER:

I kept her makeup fresh and pretty to counteract the piercing. The soft curls of her hairstyle add to this effect. Remember, when it comes to nose pierces, they leave a hole long after the piercing is gone.

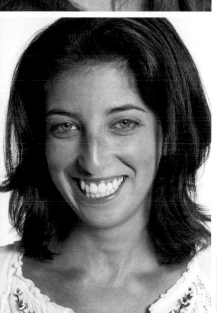
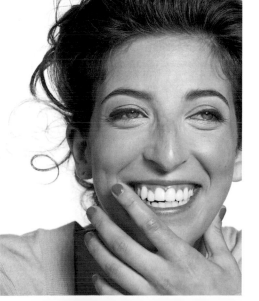

BEFORE:

Samantha has such beautiful and piercing eyes that I couldn't help but focus on them.

AFTER:

I made her eyes pop even more by using a very strong liner on her top lid. Everything else I did was in service of her eyes. I defined her brows and used a very sheer pink color on her lips so that her eyes would get all the attention. Her hair swept back adds to the effect. Her fun pink nails kept the overall look playful.

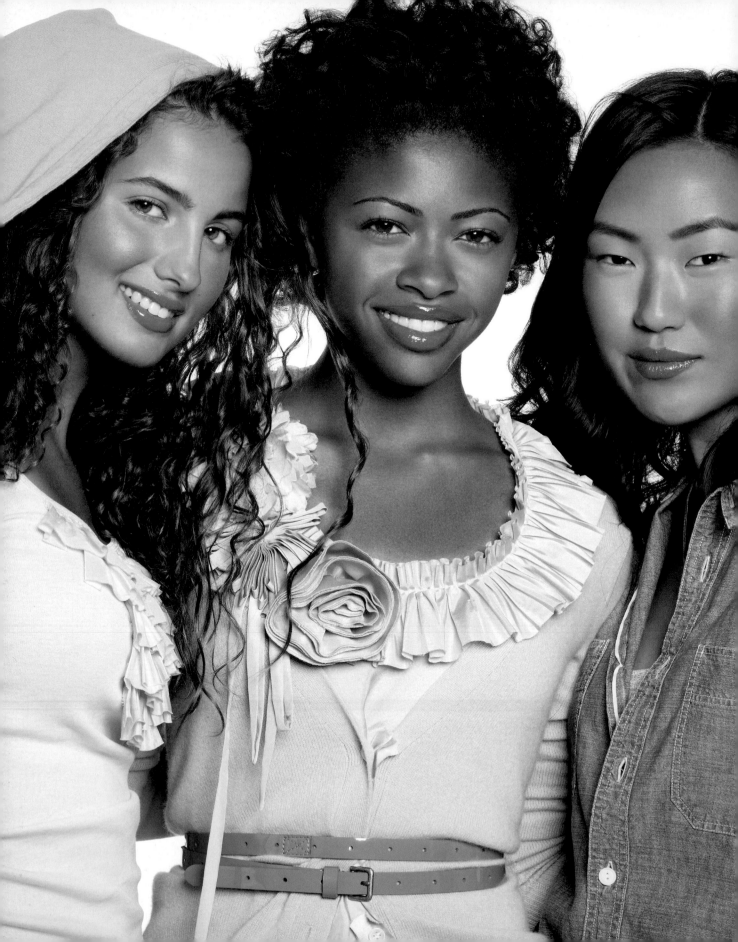

12

GLOBAL GORGEOUSNESS

Everyone's face is different, with its own special rules, quirks, and perks. No matter what color you are, you need to know what works on your skin. I don't like to generalize because everyone is unique, but there are some basic guidelines for beauty depending on whether you are African American, Latin, Asian, Middle Eastern, or a mix of any or all of the above. The most important thing for anyone to do is appreciate what you have naturally.

black skin

Many girls and women with black skin are darker across the forehead and the perimeter of the face while lighter in the middle. When it comes to foundation, often black women need two different colors of foundation to match their different skin tones. You will need to blend the colors to make the transition between them seamless.

HERE IS HOW THE TWO FOUNDATIONS SHOULD BE APPLIED:

The lighter color should go on your forehead to balance all the areas.

The darker color should go on your cheeks, the lightest part of your face.

If you are not comfortable blending two different foundations, there is another option that also creates a warmer look. Choose a tinted moisturizer that's in between the color at the center of your face and the perimeter. Use this as an overall foundation.

FINDING THE RIGHT COLOR OF FOUNDATION:

Lighter black skin looks best with a yellow-based foundation that has tints of golden orange.

Darker skin looks best with a yellow-based foundation with warm cinnamon to blue tones.

You might also use loose or pressed powder to reduce shine. If you do, get one that has yellow or orange tones if your complexion is light to medium. If you have a dark skin, find a powder with a blue tint.

HERE ARE SOME THINGS TO AVOID:

Trying to lighten skin with a lighter-colored foundation. It doesn't work.

Translucent powder, which just makes black skin look ashy.

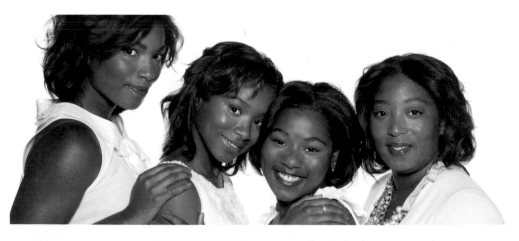

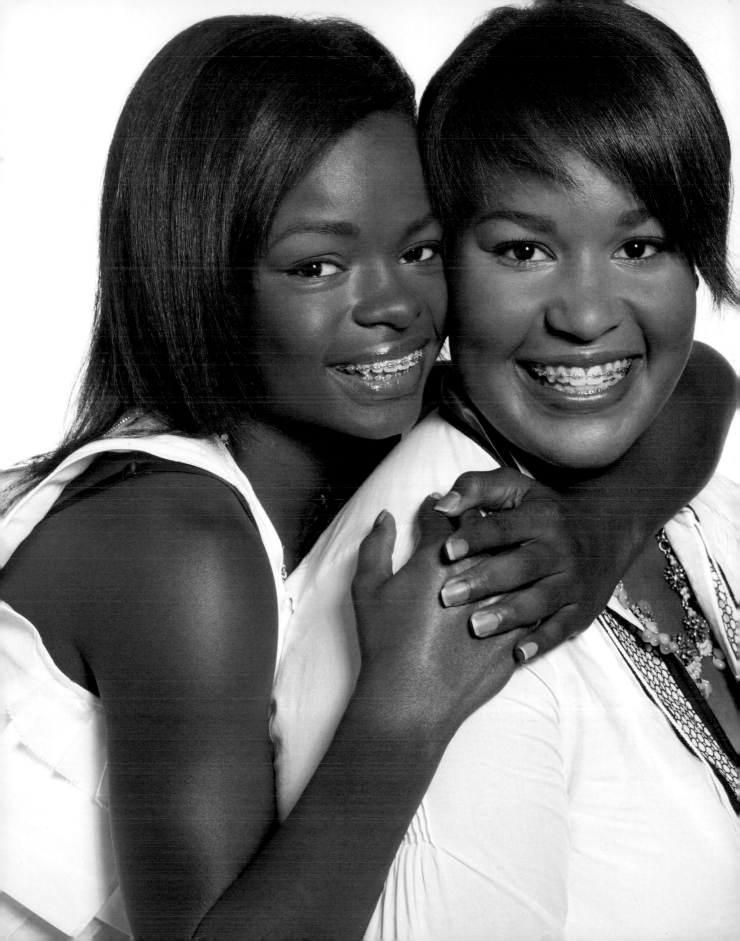

latin skin

Latina girls and women come in many skin colors, from pale to dark. No matter where you fit in the spectrum, bronzer is your best friend. Latina women, whose skin is generally a mix of golden and olive tones, tend to get a gorgeous warm glow in the summer months. But in the winter, their skin can often turn a shade of yellow-green. Bronzer is great year-round, adding even more warmth in the summer and fighting against sallow skin in the winter. A cool blush on the apples of the cheeks looks great and cuts the warmth. If you are fair, opt for a pinkish-brown bronzer. Darker skin looks best with a brownish-red bronzer.

If you need foundation to even out your overall skin tone, find a product with a yellow-gold undertone that matches your skin's natural warmth (powder should also be golden in color). One foundation warning: don't go too golden with the color or you will begin to look orange. The product should have a hint of gold, not scream it.

asian skin

A lot of Asian girls and women are concerned that using foundation with yellow tones will make their skin look too yellow. Not to worry; yellow-based foundation is the most natural looking because it's the natural tone of the skin, not only for Asian skin but also for white and black skin. It will match and enhance your complexion perfectly.

Asian women don't have a lot of darkness under their eyes, but concealer can still make a big difference and brighten the whole face.

HERE ARE SOME THINGS TO AVOID:

Pink foundation is a complete don't. It will give you an artificial look.

Skin-whitening cream is something I don't understand. Asian women have some of the most beautiful skin in the world. Don't try to change color. Spot out any dark spots, even out your skin tone, and appreciate it!

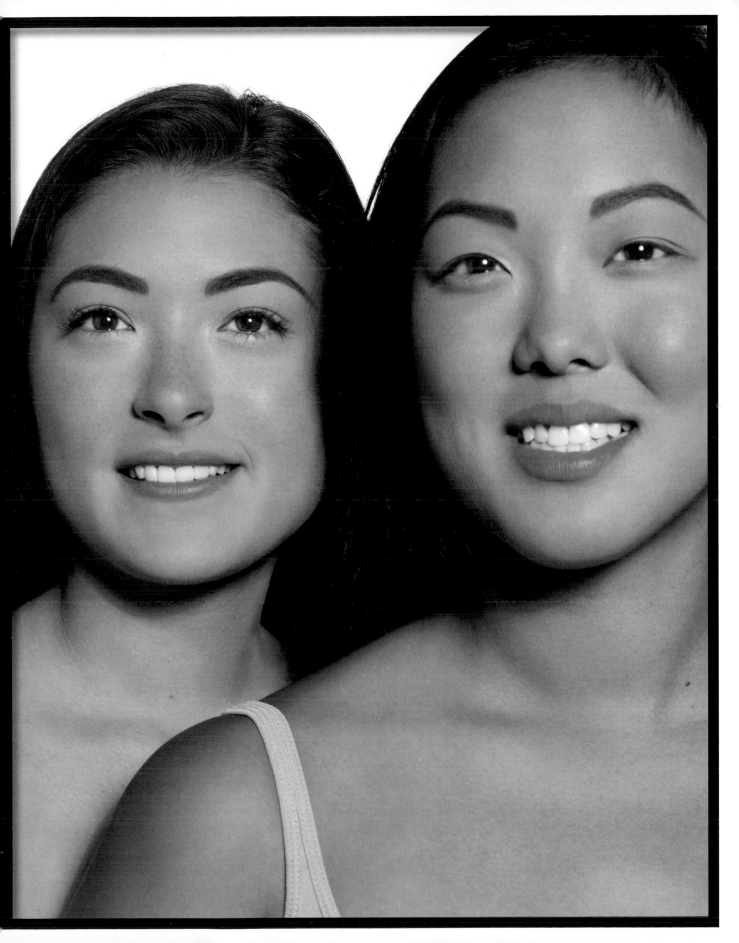

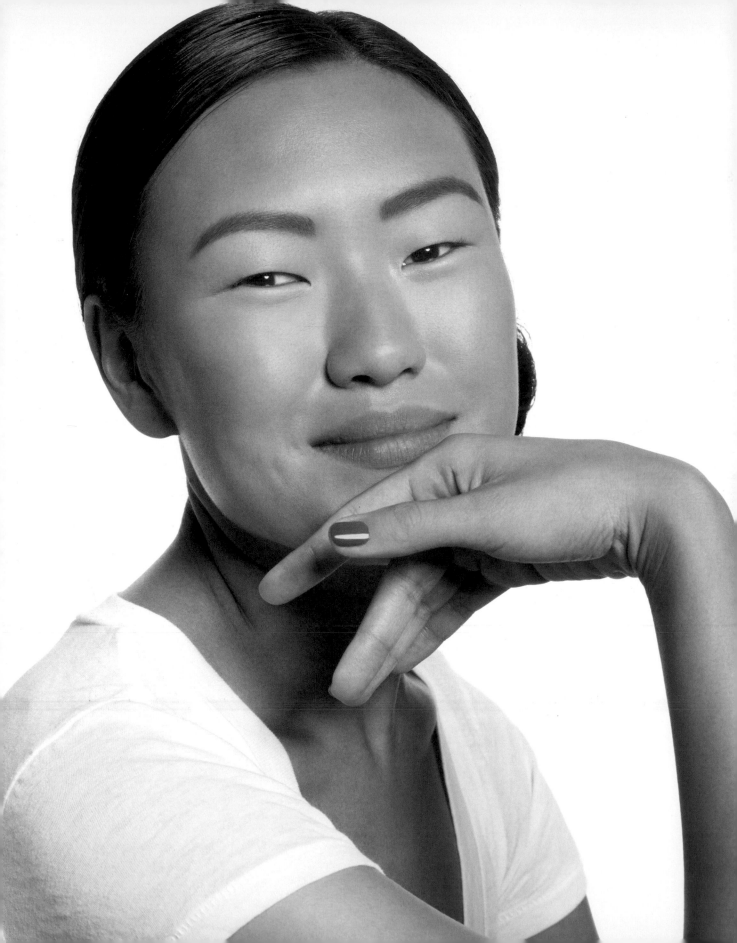

step-by-step

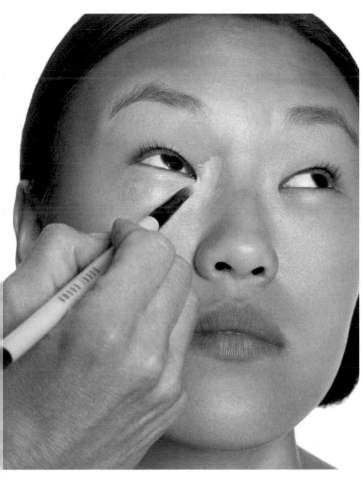

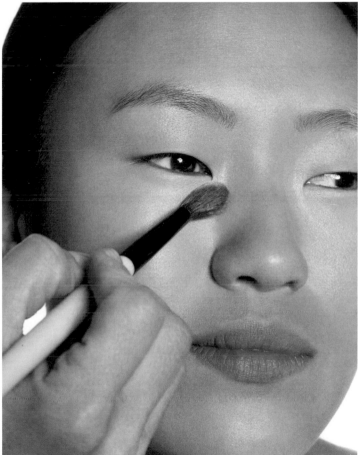

1:

Apply concealer under the eyes.

2:

Set the concealer with pale yellow powder. It's also applied on the eye lid.

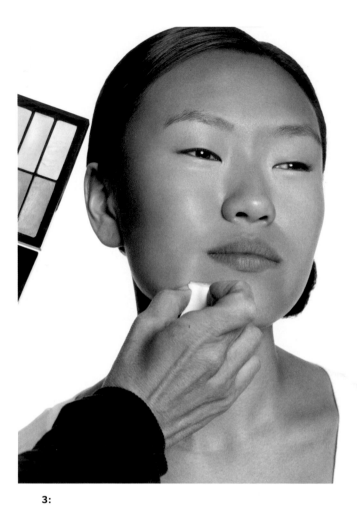

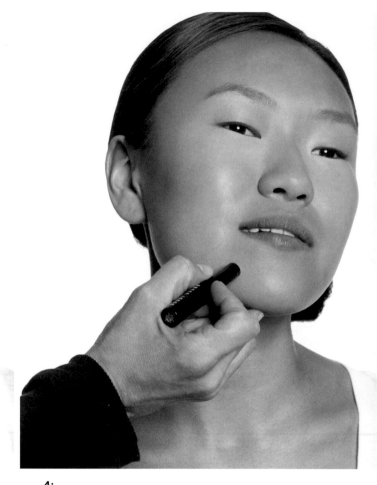

3:

Even out the skin tone with a foundation in a color that matches the skin.

4:

Any stubborn spots can be erased with the touch-up stick.

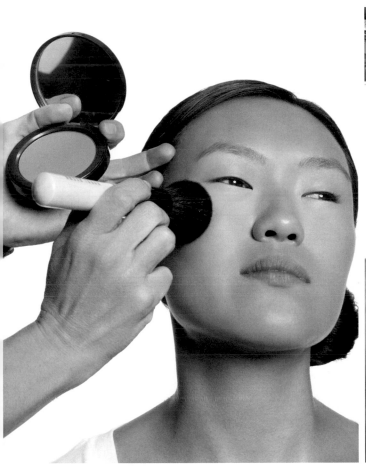

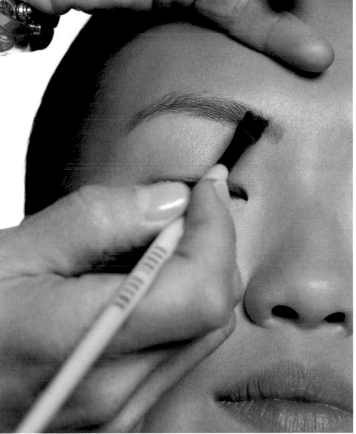

5:

Dust bronzer all over the face. Don't forget to apply it on your neck.

6:

Fill in the brows using a powder shadow with an eyebrow brush.

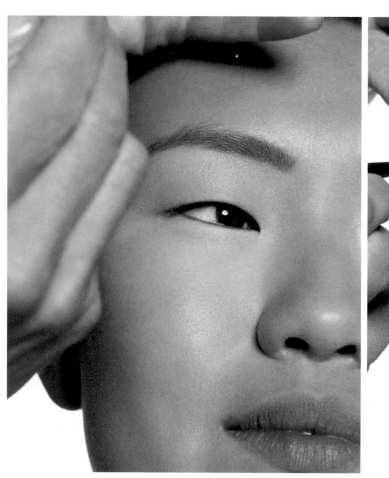

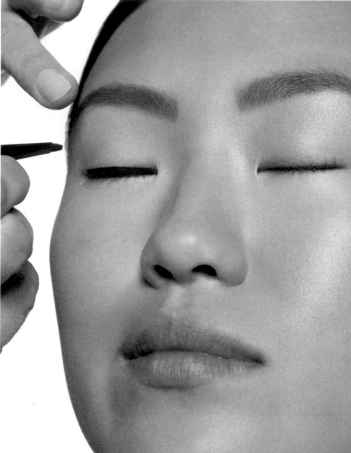

6 (CONTINUED):

When filling in your brows, you want to match the color of the hair in the brow, but also be conscious of the color of the hair on your head.

7:

Apply espresso gel liner right along the lash line with an ultrafine eyeliner brush.

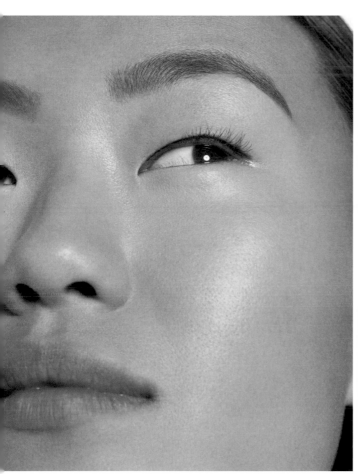
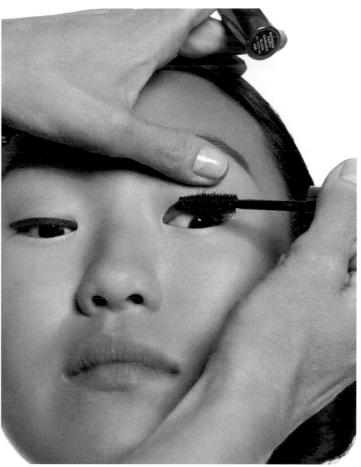

7 (CONTINUED):

Make sure the line is thick enough in order to see it when the eyes are open.

8:

Apply two or three coats of black mascara.

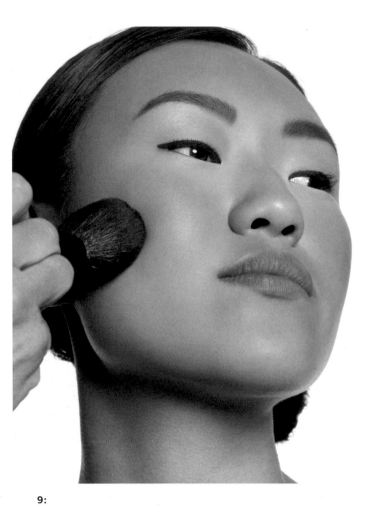

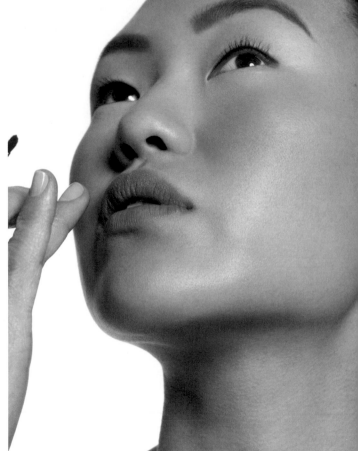

9:

Add a pop of pinkish-rose blush on the cheeks with a fluffy round blush brush.

10:

Press on a bit of natural color lipstick to enhance the natural color of the lips.

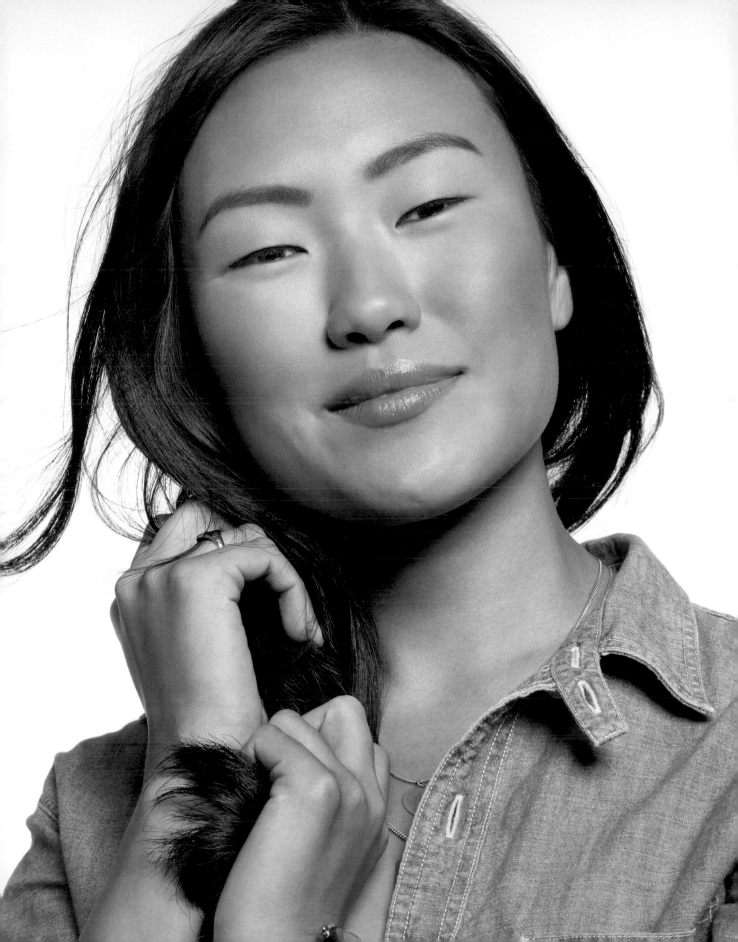

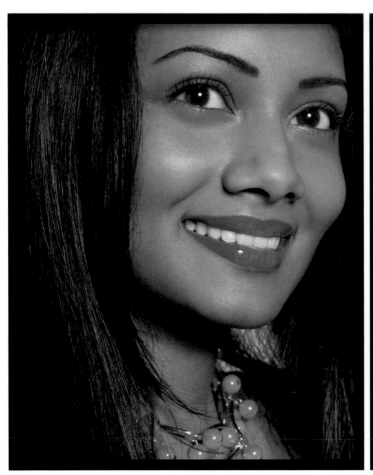

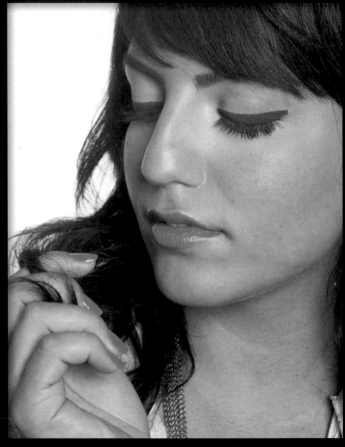

Melissa doesn't need a lot of makeup to look very exotic. I filled in her dark brows and used deep berry colors to highlight the golden tones in her skin. For Indian girls, who often have dark lips, chocolate or blackberry lipsticks are beautiful options. The pale pink or beige lip glosses that look so cool on your blond, blue-eyed friends won't work on you. If you want to go for a light color, pick one in a raisin tone.

Sunny loves looking edgy, but she also wanted to be pretty. So I kept her face really clean with the proper foundation for the yellow tones in her Middle Eastern skin. Then I added a strong eye and balanced out the whole look with a bright-pink lip. She's bold but not overdone. Her hot-pink nails and thick mod bangs add a girly light touch.

indian skin

Girls from India have amazing coloring, often with beautiful skin that has the rich-ness of dark honey. For people from this part of the world, their skin normally has a yellow-orange tone. If your skin is lighter, than you have more yellow tones. If it's darker, then there is more orange. Sometimes there are darker tones on the fore-head that you have to balance out. But the hardest part of evening out the skin is dealing with the darkness around the eyes. Indian girls often have a greenish, purple tint not just underneath their eyes but also on the eyelids, in the corners and underneath. That's why it's important not to simply apply a dark eye shadow, which will make the eyes recede. First, lighten up the eye area with a corrector and concealer. It works well to have two correctors in two different colors (try one that's pinkish and another in a peachy color). Use a lighter color in the inner eye area and the other color on top and underneath. Most important, experiment with your products until you get the results you want. There is not one magic formula. But familiarizing yourself with how makeup affects your skin tone will answer your biggest skin questions.

middle eastern skin

Girls of Middle Eastern descent often have the most alluring eyes. Darkness under those gorgeous eyes can be an issue. Use a corrector under your concealer to brighten the under-the-eye area. You might have to layer a few correctors before you get it right. Begin with peach or pink, and then layer yellow concealer on top. To match your skin tone, try a yellow-toned foundation with a bit of orange.

Middle Eastern eyes look amazing with black liner. Don't use liner that is lighter than mahogany. Give your cheeks color with blush in deep rose and pink shades. You can keep lips neutral to balance the strong liner. To layer on the drama, go very pale or try a deep-red stain on the lips.

multiethnic skin

Girls with parents of different ethnicities have that incredible beauty that comes from mixing skin types, eye shapes, and hair textures. Sometimes it can be hard because you might not look like your dad or your mom, so you don't have an immediate beauty role model to turn to. But you are lucky because your look is totally unique.

Often a big issue for girls who come from different ethnicities is figuring out how to deal with all the different colors in their skin. See what I did with Rachel, on the following pages, who is so beautifully blended in her own unique tone.

step-by-step

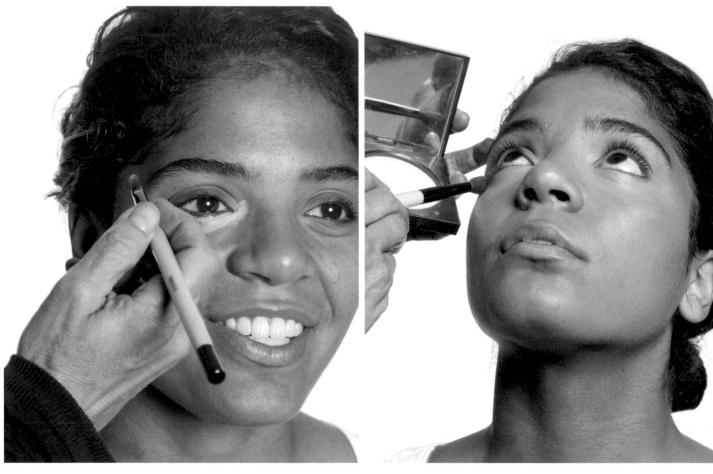

1:

Apply peach corrector under the eyes. Start where you need it the most (where the skin is the darkest). Usually that's at the inner corner of the eye. Blend the product under the eye completely with a brush or your finger.

2:

Set the corrector with yellow powder, which is also applied all over the lids to act as an eye base.

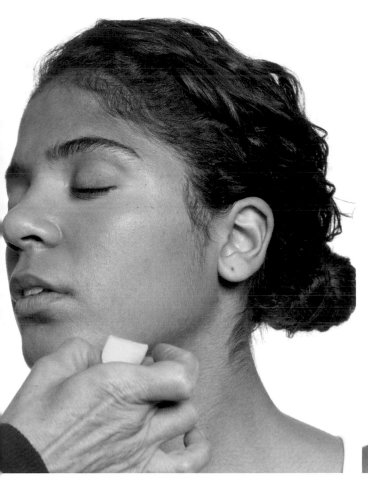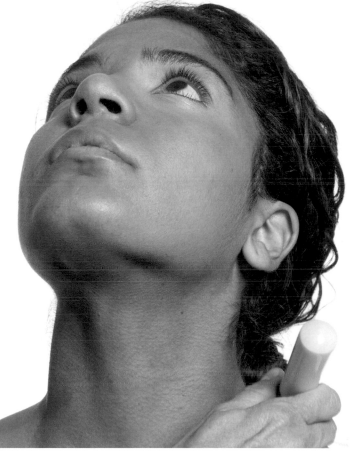

3:

To get a foundation that's right for all the colors in your face, start with a foundation that works on your cheeks, but make sure it also works on your forehead. (On Rachel, using a sponge, I applied a golden foundation that disappeared into her skin and evened out her different pigments.)

4:

Swipe bronzer lightly on the neck to even out the skin tone. If you have oily skin, you can brush powder over your foundation.

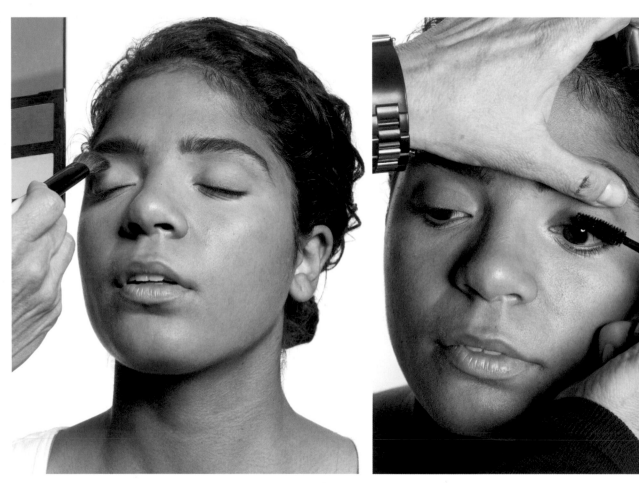

5:

Choose a base shadow that is warm to blend into the skin tone. Layer shadows such as toast and cocoa to create definition.

6:

Apply two or three coats of mascara.

Plum blush gives the cheeks a healthy glow. A gloss in pink beige is the finishing touch.

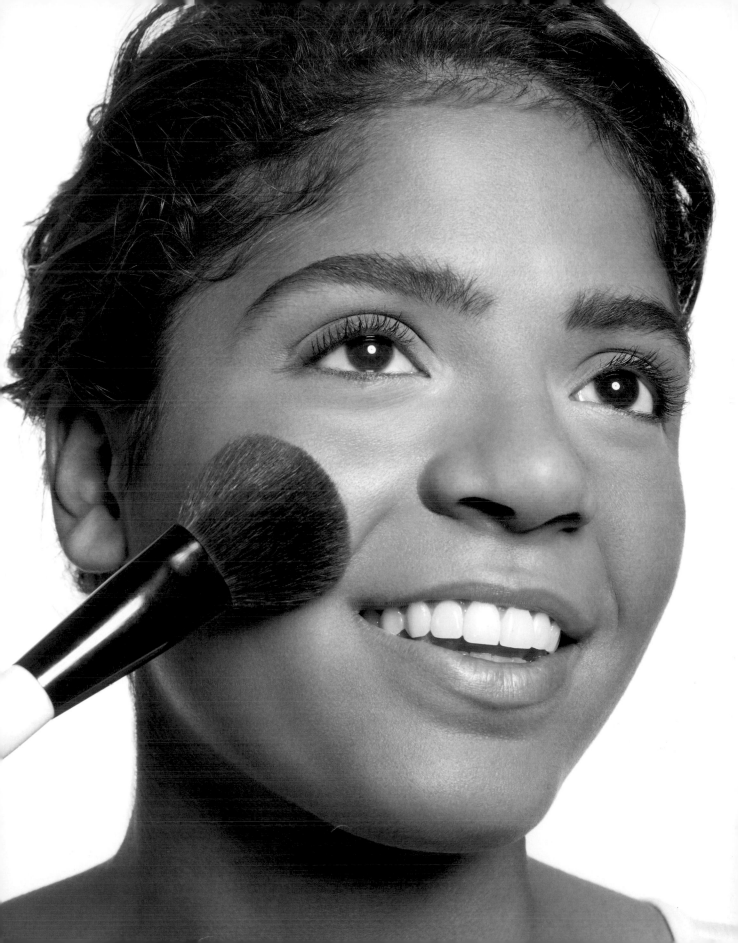

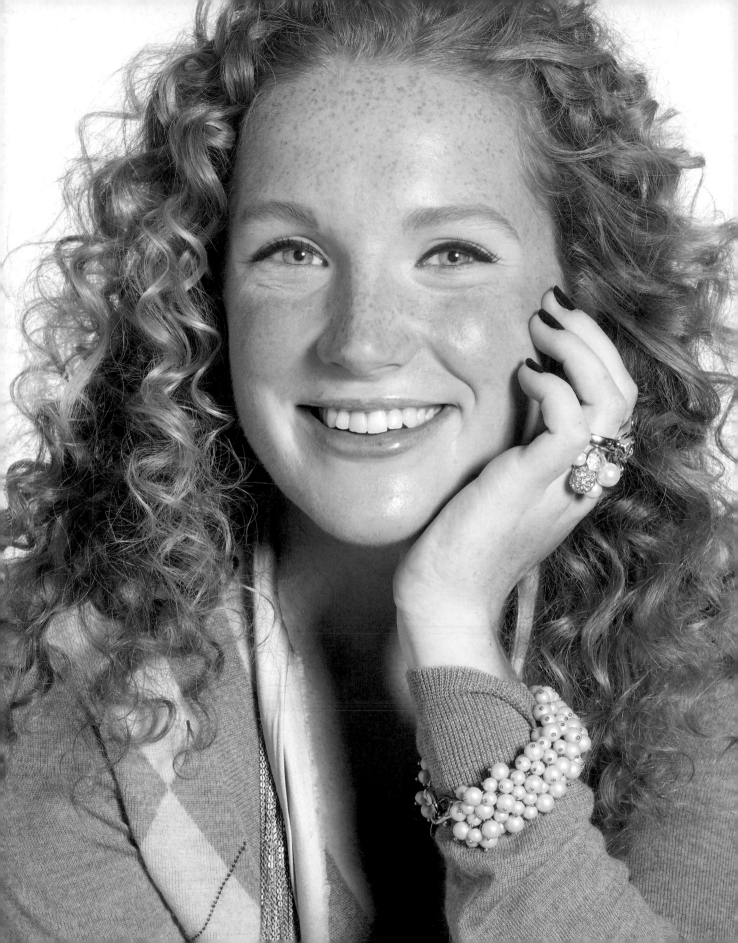

13

TOTAL STYLE

My style is all about simplicity and comfort and tailoring. I love classic things, and at 5 feet tall, I look better in clothes that are cut for my body. That doesn't mean my style is boring. I'm always going for the unexpected when I get dressed. I would rather pair a stack of sparkly bracelets with jeans than a fancy dress because the contrast is what makes it interesting. You've got to mix it up.

The best way to develop your own sense of style is to look at what other girls are wearing on the street or in school. That might sound like a contradiction, but style is all about inspiration. When I was a teen, we didn't have that many celebrity magazines or Web sites to follow the latest fashions. So I used to look at my girlfriends. There was Lynn, the coolest-looking girl, who would throw on these hippie clothes that looked amazing on her, but not on me. Then there was the girl who wore a perfect combat jacket, sending me on a mission to the army and navy store to find the same one for myself. In a lot of ways, we were lucky not to be bombarded with images of celebs. Without a closet full of designer-label clothes and a team of stylists, you can't get the same look.

The sources of inspiration exploded around me when I left Chicago and arrived in New York City as a young makeup artist. I was working in the fashion industry with the most talented editors, models, photographers, and stylists in the world. I studied them hard as I went through a wild period of experimentation. I went through my Madonna moment and my Joan Jett period until I slowed down and started to see how the really cool stylists would wear a certain pair of slouchy loafers, low-top Converse sneakers, or a big masculine watch (all items that are now staples in my wardrobe). It took a while to hone in on a style that not only looks good but also feels good.

YOU CAN FIND STYLE INSPIRATION EVERYWHERE, FROM MAGAZINES TO GIRLFRIENDS.

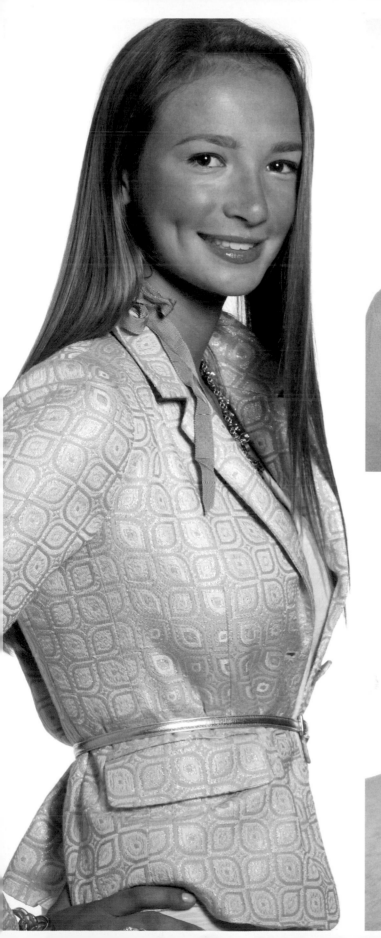
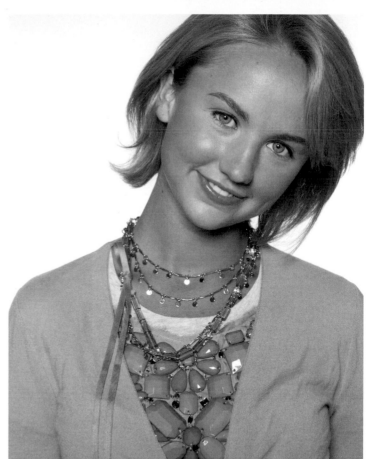
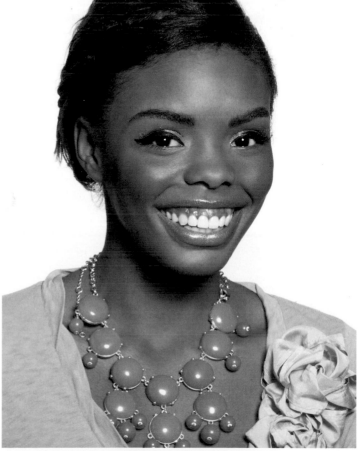

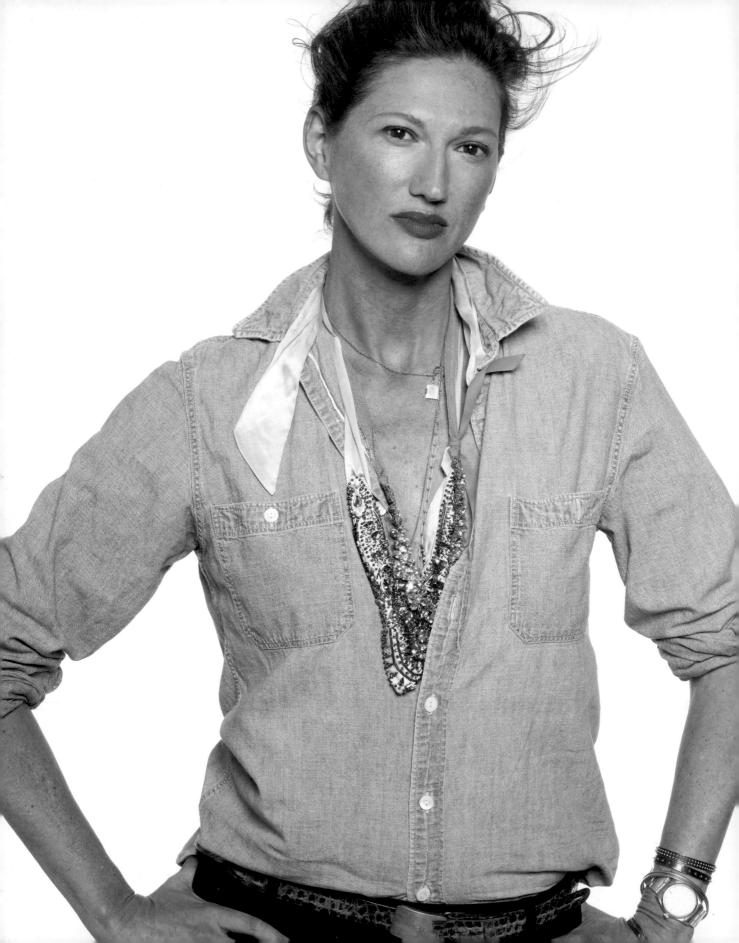

INTERVIEW: JENNA LYONS
TOP STYLIST TELLS ALL

Jenna Lyons is one of the most amazing people working in fashion today. As creative director of J. Crew, she's in charge of everything from what clothes are sold to how the stores look to the models you see in the catalogs. That's a huge job, and she does it well. But the coolest thing about Jenna is her style: she's super-eclectic. She can take the basics or something that might have come out of grandma's closet and make it look new again. She's further proof that classic doesn't have to be boring.

When did you first get interested in fashion?

When I was in seventh grade, I was 6 feet tall and didn't fit into anything. So I got a sewing machine and a subscription to *Vogue* and decided to make a basic skirt. I was so completely unable to find anything in the stores that fit me that it was pure desperation. I remember the fabric exactly—it was a watermelon pattern. It was hard being really tall. I was gawky and not pretty. I had really frizzy hair, and my mom didn't let me wear makeup. On top of that, I have a genetic disorder so my legs were covered in scars. I made a long skirt to cover my scars, but I was terrified to wear it to school. I didn't have a lot of friends. Kids can be cruel. I was terrified of everyone and everything. When I wore the skirt to school, someone said she loved it. I felt my walk change. To have someone compliment me on something I wore was life altering. It made me want to do more. That was the start, but it was a long road to becoming confident.

What was your style like when you were a teen?

It was a funny mix of California and East Coast. I lived on the West Coast, but I had a stylish East Coast grandmother. She would send me kilts with gold buttons. I'll never forget wearing a wool kilt with a graphic rock-concert T shirt for the first day of school in California! No one wore that stuff. Then there were the '80s, which were a total disaster, but I came out of it.

How did you break into the fashion industry?

I found that whenever I wore something I made, people would ask me where I got it. That was so rewarding and exciting, it made me want to do more. There was no *Project Runway* back then. I did my research and found out about Parsons [a New York City school, which has a renowned fashion department] through an art teacher. I applied, got in, and after graduation worked at Donna Karan. I started at J. Crew nineteen years ago as an assistant to an assistant to an assistant.

What's the best part of your job?

I love that every day is completely different. Today we are talking about our holiday shoot in Chile—the locations, how much snow we want to have, and getting the models on a horse ranch. Then I'm going to a new kids' store that we are opening. Later I have meetings to work on specialty shoes, jewelry, and colors for fall. I wouldn't be the best person behind a desk.

What does your closet look like?

My closet is insane. It is an entire room in the house. I have two floor-to-ceiling shoe racks that are 6 feet wide and 11 feet high and filled to the gills. The clothes are organized by color, then type. I give away a lot. I am a huge giver-away-er. If I buy five new pairs of shoes, I give five away. My husband is a little bit over it. I get dressed starting with my shoes. I don't know why I do that. It became a sport with my three-year-old son, Beckett, who chooses the shoes.

How can girls find their own great style? What are some of your secrets to experimenting successfully?

The most important thing is to listen and repeat. If someone pays you a compliment because you look great, take note. If you are wearing your hair back or you have a bright red lip on, and someone says you look great, wear that again. It is not about wearing the latest trend. I can't wear a lot of things. I don't like my legs, so I don't wear shorts or short skirts. But I am really tall, so I look really good in skinny pants and high heels. It is about playing with your best strengths.

Where do you get your inspiration from when coming up with outfits?

Everything. Blogs. Cool people on the street. I love people watching. If it were an Olympic sport, I would be a gold medalist. I am addicted to magazines. It is like a sickness.

From the sounds of your closet, you do a lot of shopping. Any advice?

Buying things on sale is dangerous. It encourages people to buy things that aren't great for them because they are cheap. You are not going on gut love, but on price. That's not a great way to build a wardrobe. Buy fewer things, but make them amazing clothes you love.

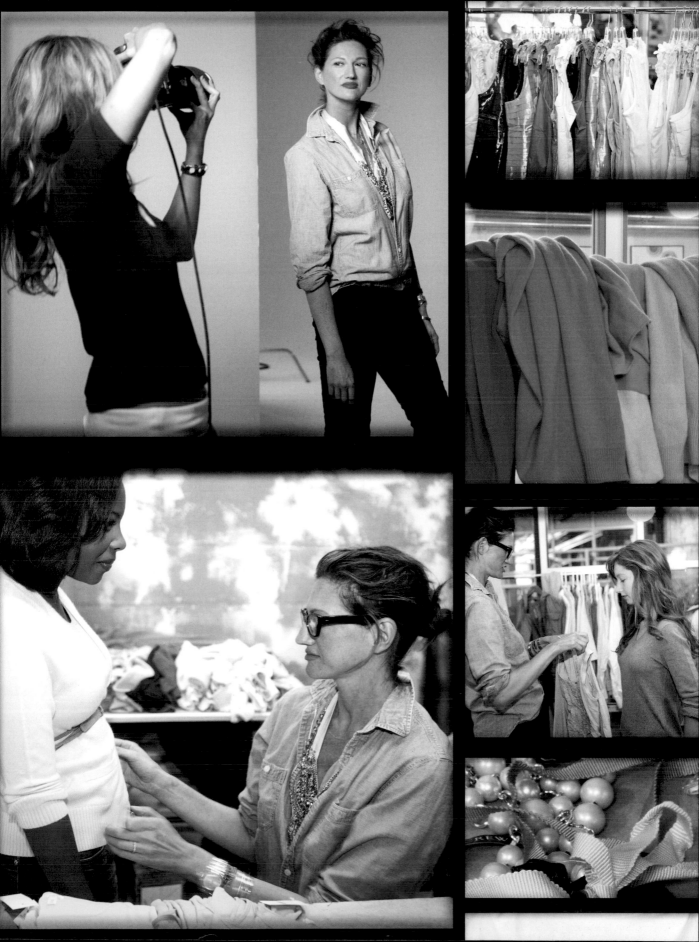

What are some clothing items you think are worth spending more money on?

Shoes. Especially if you are younger and getting ready to go into the workforce. There's nothing more tragic than a really ratty pair of shoes. Another mark of taste and style is a watch. A cell phone is not a timepiece. There is a certain elegance for a girl or boy to own a watch.

How can accessories change a look?

Pairing clothes with completely opposite accessories can extend the life of your wardrobe. One of my favorite tricks is to take a white, cotton summer dress and bring it into the fall with black tights, boots, and a blazer. The contrast can look really great. Then in summer you can wear the same dress with bare legs and flip-flops.

What's your advice to someone who wants to change her style?

Thrift stores are an awesome place to try new stuff. Give away a lot of your clothes, and get into someone else's closet. Mix up your clothes with your best friends'. It can be fun. Especially when you are young, you have time to change it up.

How would you define real style?

Even magazines for kids are very retouched. It is very intimidating and can make it hard to understand how to represent yourself. Style is not just about looking good. It's about sharing yourself. When you have great style, it can mean a beautiful smile and a great handshake. If you walk over to someone you don't know at a party and say hi, that's stylish. If your internal style is amazing, then what you wear will look even better, no matter what you're wearing.

JENNA + BOBBI'S QUICK TIPS FOR SUPER STYLE

TIP NUMBER ONE:
LITTLE THINGS MEAN A LOT

TINY TWEAKS TO AN OUTFIT CAN COMPLETELY CHANGE IT UP. IT COULD BE A BELT AROUND THE OUTSIDE OF A JACKET, UNBUTTONING A PAIR OF PANTS AT THE TOP, OR TURNING A COLLAR UP. TAKE AN OUTFIT THAT ISN'T WORKING AND SEE IF LITTLE ADJUSTMENTS CAN TURN IT AROUND.

TIP NO. 3: TAKE A PAGE FROM GIRLS ON THE STREET

Fashion magazines aren't the only source for new ideas. There are probably women you see every day with amazing style. Don't be afraid to learn from them.

TIP NO. 5: DON'T BE A BARGAIN HUNTER

It's great to be economical. But spending a lot of money on stuff you probably won't wear just because it's on sale is a serious waste. Go for quality not quantity. Buy one, two or, maybe if you're lucky, three beautiful pieces that make you crazy and forget the rest of the stuff. If you have your eye on a piece of clothing that you can't afford all season and get it when it goes on sale, you've hit the fashion jackpot.

FOLLOW YOUR SHAPE
TIP NO. 2:

Pay attention to your shape and who you are and don't worry about what everyone else is doing. If skinny jeans don't suit you, that's OK. There's another trend around the corner that does.

TIP NUMBER 4: COLOR GUARD

If you have darker skin, it is anything goes when it comes to color. If you have very pale skin, be careful of colors that match your hair. The exception is pale brunettes, who can wear and look great in brown.

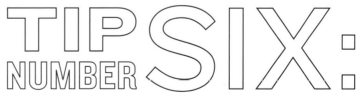
TIP NUMBER SIX:
BE INTERESTING

MAKE YOUR STYLE CHOICES SURPRISING. PEARLS ARE GREAT ON A YOUNG GIRL. MAKE THOSE DEMURE PEARLS REALLY SAY SOMETHING BY PAIRING THEM WITH A JEAN JACKET, SLOUCHY PANTS, AND A T-SHIRT.

TIP NUMBER SEVEN: HAVE FUN
THERE ARE NO REALLY IMPORTANT STYLE RULES WHEN YOU ARE YOUNG.

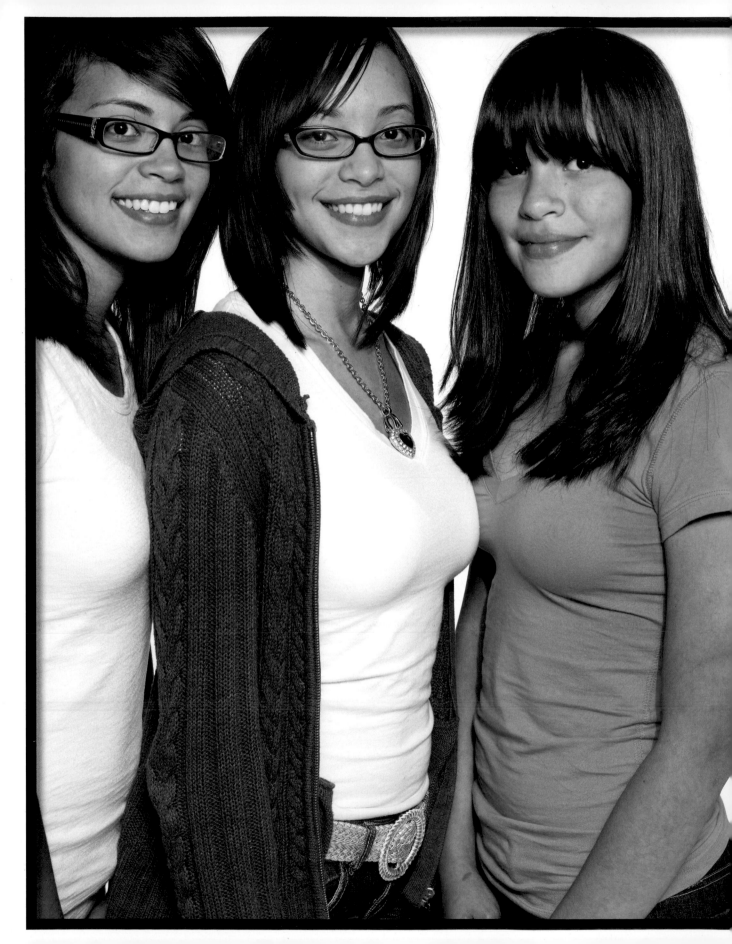

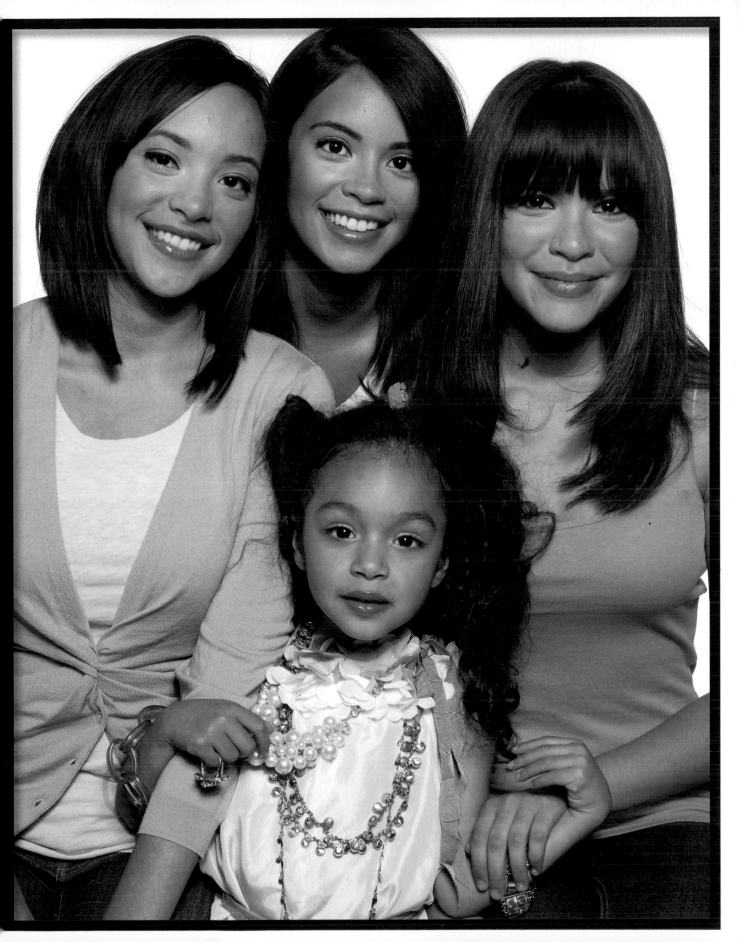

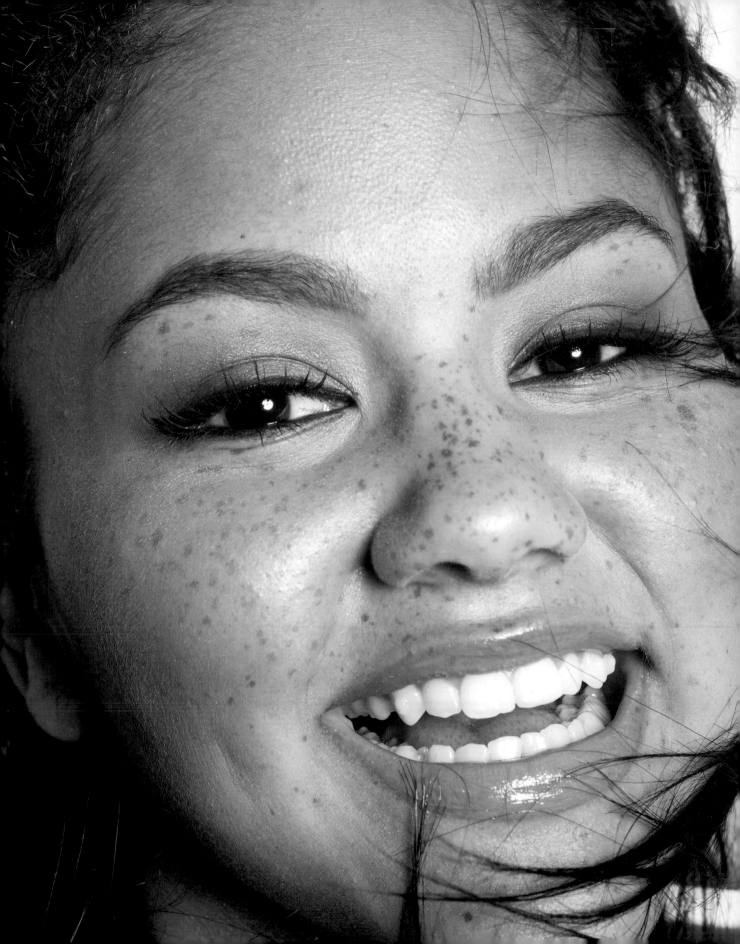

14

PARTY TIME

Everyone loves dressing up. It is fun and glamorous and makes you feel special. Whether it's for a big party, school dance, or just a family celebration, it's a good time to experiment. Sometimes the preparation is even more fun than actually going to the event.

bar and bat mitzvahs

This is usually a time that girls wear makeup out—twelve to thirteen is a good time to start experimenting with lip gloss, mascara, and maybe a bit of pale shimmer shadow on the lid. I know many girls who buy dresses for the first time (hello, jocks). You have to dress up for temple and most parties. My advice here is go simple. Casual chic is the key (most parties include dancing, so wear comfy shoes, although most girls wind up kicking them off). Don't worry—soon enough you'll be wearing fancier dresses.

quinceañera, sweet sixteen, and birthdays

Girls do begin to experiment with more makeup and grown-up dresses. It is amazing to me how gorgeous girls look when they let themselves take the next step in party dressing. The trick here is not to dress too revealing and wear too much makeup. (Remember: if you have it, you don't have to go over the top to show it! Everyone sees it anyway.)

prom and formals

Girls wait their whole lives for their big school dance. It is like their own personal fashion show with a pretty (and sometimes too sexy) dress, a hairdresser, makeup (for some, even an artist to do their makeup), jewelry, and totally awesome shoes. It is sometimes a shock to see the sporty girls look like Beyoncé or Jennifer Lopez. You can totally transform for the night. Cinderella meets *Vogue*.

I do see some girls make huge mistakes that take partying too far with revealing dresses that are more bothersome and uncomfortable than flattering. It is better to be more safe than sorry. Bring a wrap just in case. Be open and have fun.

REMEMBER WHAT'S MOST IMPORTANT...

HAVE FUN!

PROM PREP TIMELINE
GABI + BOBBI

To get inspired, check out how Gabi prepared for her big night celebrating.

A Year Before

GABI: I knew exactly what I was going to wear a whole year before. I was going through my grandma's closet and came across this black lace frock that she had made for her engagement party. I tried it on and knew it would look good if I wore a simple black slip and the right shoes. I asked her, and she let me have it.

BOBBI: Gabi's style inspiration came to her really naturally. If you need to work at it a little more, about six months before your big event, look in magazines and talk to your friends to see what they're thinking of wearing. Don't forget a very important source of ideas: your own closet. Shop your own closet by digging deep. You might find that ugly dress of your sister's that unleashes your inner fashion designer. Cut it. Pin it. See what happens. Whether you make your dress or buy it, don't sacrifice comfort for glamour. These days there are plenty of dresses and shoes that fill both categories.

Three Months Before

GABI: I started thinking about how to wear the lace dress, which is very complex. I knew I couldn't wear too many accessories. The dress speaks for itself. But I wanted to wear a simple shoe with an open toe, a cocktail ring, and a simple necklace. I am a big jewelry person, so I looked through my own collection and found a faux diamond and pearl cocktail ring from a local store. Then I borrowed a diamond necklace that belongs to my mother.

BOBBI: Try on your dress for your family and friends. Given the thumbs-up—move on to the fun stuff. Shoes, jewelry, and just the right tiny purse.

A Month Before

GABI: I asked Cody if he wanted to go to the prom. He is a friend of mine, and I thought he would be a fun date. I like him as a person and think he is a funny guy. I wanted to go with someone I felt comfortable with and that I would have an enjoyable time with. No drama.

BOBBI: Finding a makeup artist should be a lot less stressful than finding a date. Start by asking around. Word of mouth is definitely the way to go. Book an appointment at a nearby salon or a makeup counter at a local department store. Ask for someone who specializes in teen beauty, prom makeup, or smoky eyes. Make sure you ask the price of an application. Stores often will offer a free trial, while makeup artists charge a nominal amount for an application. Prices vary, so always ask first.

If you do your own makeup (and why not? You've got all the info on how to do it) and are looking for some new ideas, you can get advice from online makeup artists. Many makeup companies have this service on their Web sites: simply type in what you look like or attach a photo, and you'll get color and application recommendations. Makeup artists are always sharing tips with each other. It never hurts to get a fresh perspective.

Make sure you take a photo to see how the makeup looks. Photographs are a big part of any special event, so you want to see how the makeup looks on camera. Take note of how long and well the makeup lasts. Walk around the mall, eat dinner, and check out how you look before you go to bed.

Two Weeks Before

GABI: I shopped for my shoes and found a beautiful pair of sling-backs in cream. I also figured out how to wear my hair and booked an appointment with a stylist. I knew it had to be up. So I decided on a low bun with a braid in it. I usually wear my hair in a low bun because it suits me. The braid was something I thought would look cute.

BOBBI: Book your beauty appointments (try to make your hair and nail appointments before 3 P.M. so you have plenty of time to get ready). Buy any products that you have fallen in love with. During your trial, you might have discovered a great under-eye concealer or gel liner. Let whatever makeup creates the biggest wow be your guide for touch-ups that night. If red lips are your focus, bring along your lipstick. If a shimmer brick is what makes you happy, have one in your purse. If you have oily skin, pick up some blotting papers or a small compact to reduce shine at the party.

Three Days Before

GABI: I painted my toenails red.

One Day Before

GABI: I got a manicure with my friend. I usually do it myself, but if I have extra money I'll have them done professionally. It is part of the presentation and gives the look closure. I chose red as my color. I love red nails. I think it is really chic. It is something you can wear any season, and it will always look good. It's classic. I love classic.

BOBBI: Get a good night's sleep (if you can).

Afternoon of Event

GABI: We were allowed to leave school at noon, so I went home for a little bit and ate a lunch of salad with my mom. After lunch, I went to Bobbi's studio, and she did my makeup. She started off with a foundation. Then she did my eyes with black liner, mascara, and a light shimmer on my lid. She also put on a little bit of blush. Originally, I wanted to wear a red lip, but it wouldn't have worked with a strong eye. We decided a strong eye would be best with light lip gloss. Then I went to my hair appointment right after, about 3 P.M.

BOBBI: If you are doing your own makeup, give yourself plenty of time. You don't want your mother calling out for you to hurry up while you have eye shadow flaking down your face. Make getting ready for the evening an event instead of a chore. Invite friends over, and put on your favorite music. It will help keep your hand steady even as your stomach gets fluttery.

Right Before the Event

GABI: I went home and I watched TV for a little bit. In my clutch I put my phone, a little vial of the Prada perfume I wear, lip gloss, and my prom tickets. That was it. I had a Diet Coke before I left. I love Diet Coke, and it happened to be in my fridge.

BOBBI: Eat a little something so you don't pass out from exhaustion or nerves at the party. Have a snack that includes protein and carbs, like a turkey sandwich on seven-grain bread or a low-sugar energy bar.

At the Prom!

GABI: I had fun. It wasn't something that I stressed out about, but I loved getting dressed up, and having Bobbi do my makeup was really incredible. I hadn't done anything like that before. Going with Cody was definitely a good idea. It was very relaxed. There was no pressure. We were just friends at an event hanging out. My favorite part of the whole night was arriving and seeing what everyone else was wearing after planning for months or, in my case, a year.

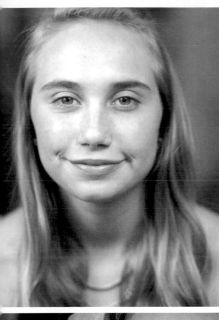
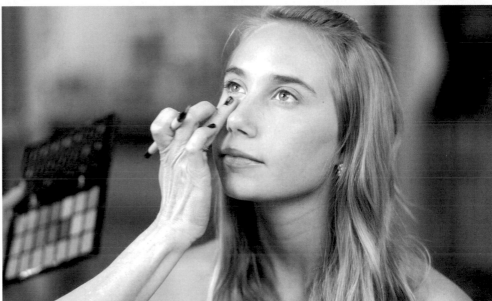
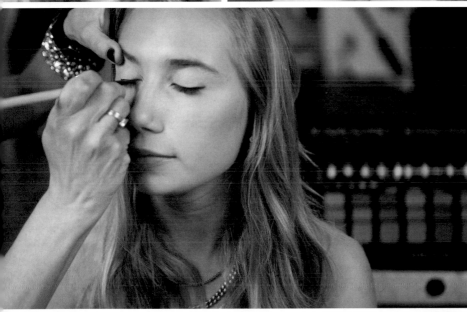
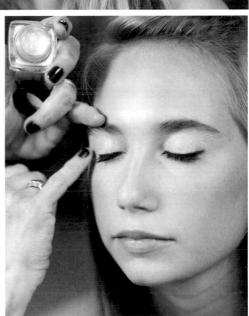
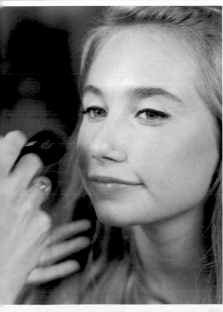
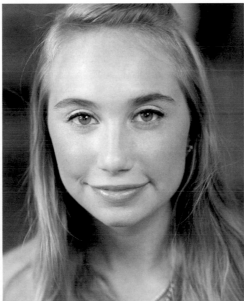
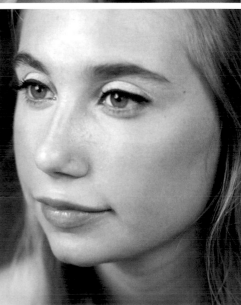

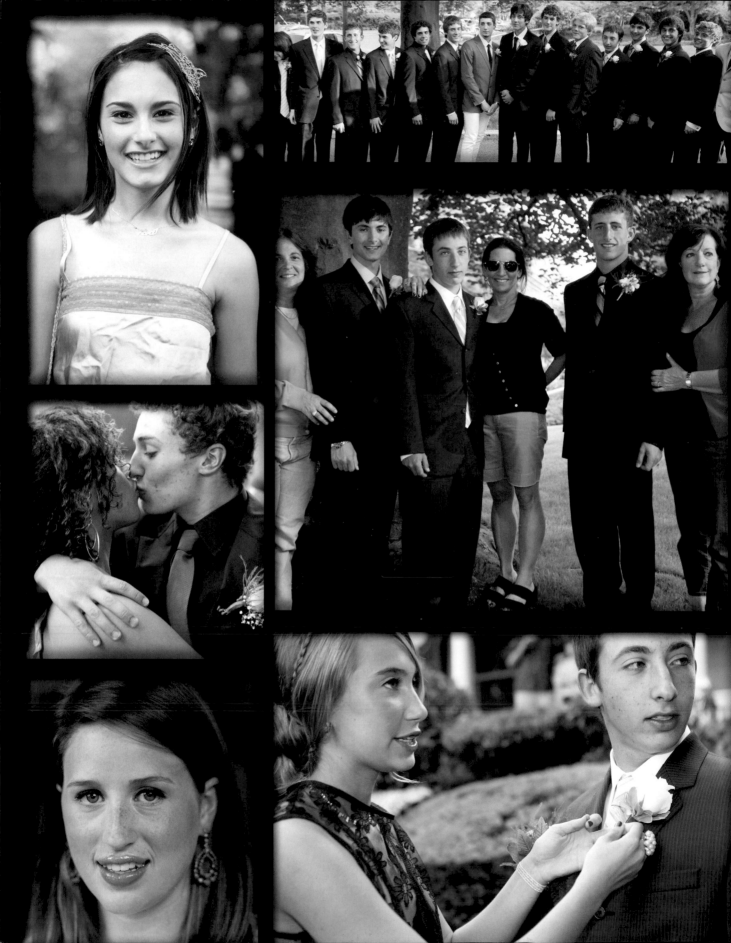

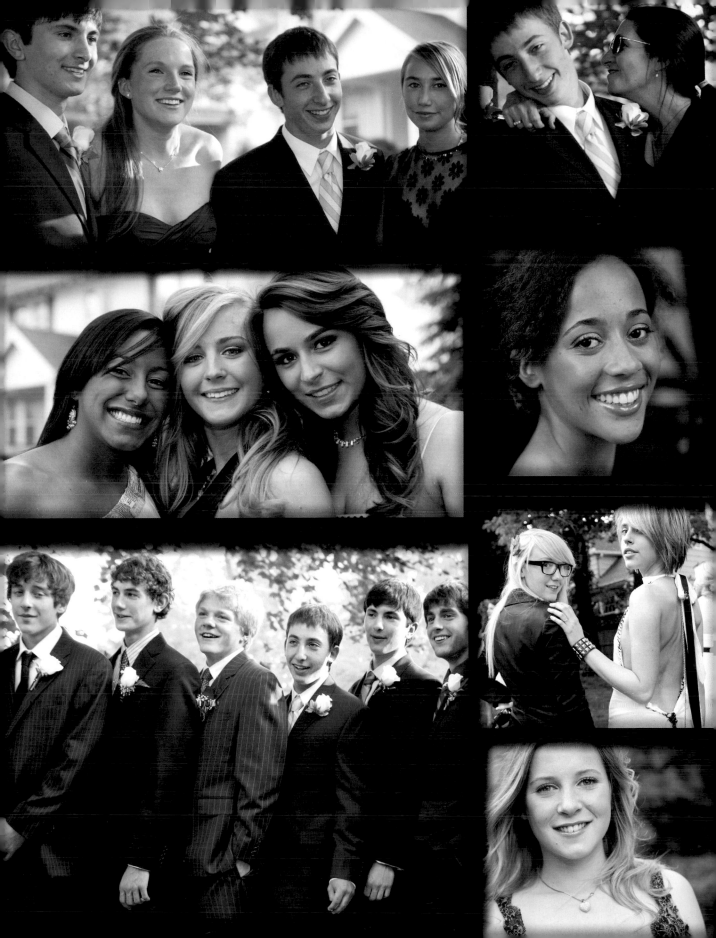

do-good beauty party

A girl's sweet sixteen or her *quinceañera* will be a night full of friends, fun, and memories. But you can make these events or any birthday party extra special by giving back. Find a way to add a charity element like the girls mentioned below.

DRESS WITH DIGNITY

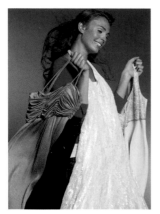

Christina was inspired to create her charity, Dresses with Dignity, which donates formal dresses to less-fortunate girls for big events like the prom, after going through her own closet. She looked at all the dresses she had worn only once and realized she could put them to good use. "There was such an abundance," she says. Christina, who has a passion for fashion, spent the better part of that spring e-mailing, working the phones, and talking to local media to get the word out about her cause. Her goal was to collect 100 dresses, but she said she would have been happy if she could get even a handful. Christina wound up surpassing her goal and brought in 156 dresses for girls who couldn't afford to shop for their prom (she also got three drycleaners to donate their services). "I had to stay focused and had to give up doing a lot of other stuff," Christina says. "In the end, it was worth it. I realized that even a dress can make such a difference in a person's life."

A VERY SWEET SIXTEEN

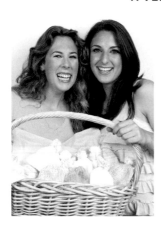

Hanna wanted the sweet-sixteen makeup party I threw for her at my studio to be a true reflection of her personality. She invited all her friends, ordered big platters of sushi (her favorite food), played great tunes (she's an insane Jonas Brothers fan), and, of course, experimented with tons of makeup. Hanna and her friends love makeup so they were thrilled to have professionals give them makeovers. They also got to create their own lip gloss with pigments and sparkles to channel their inner Bobbi. And let's not forget about the goody bags filled with cool new products. But there was one more aspect of Hanna present at the party: her charity, Gifts of Knits. Last winter, Hanna—who has participated in a mother-daughter knitting group for the last two years—wanted to do something for other people. "I had an idea. When my friend Amanda, who is also in the group, and I were born in the same hospital, we were given little knitted caps. We found out that our mothers loved these hats and kept them all these years," Hanna says. "By now we were pretty good with basic knitting techniques, so we decided to make these little baby hats for charity." They contacted a local hospital, which was in need of newborn hats. So Hanna and Amanda started knitting and delivered the first batch to the maternity ward personally. At her sweet-sixteen party, Hanna asked her friends to donate yarn so that she and Amanda could keep knitting.

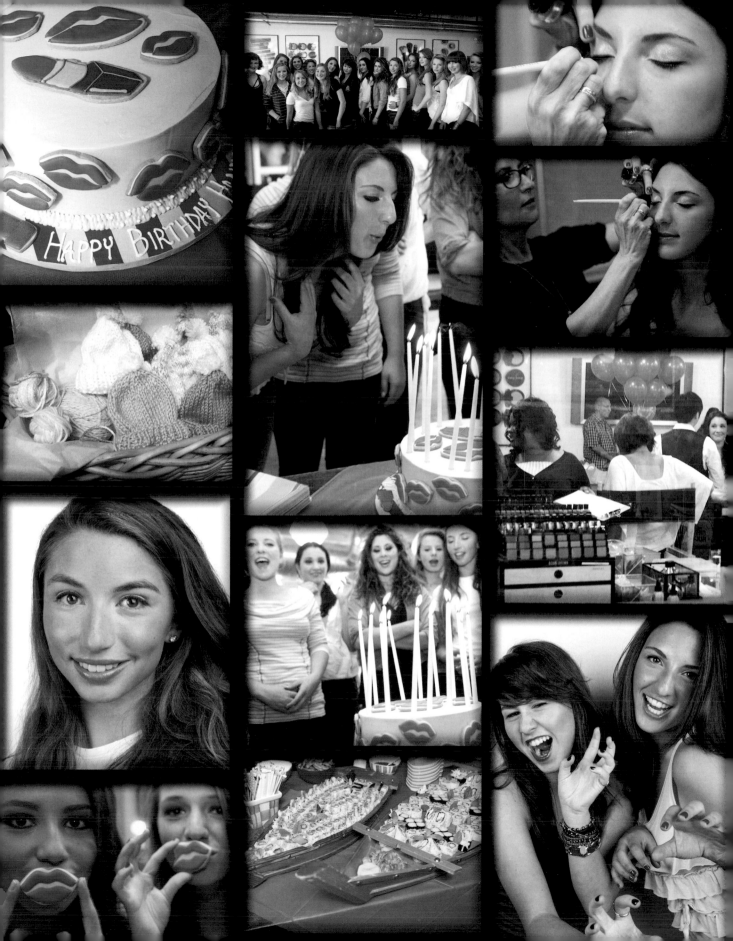

PLAY WITH YOUR LOOK

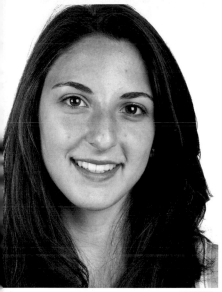

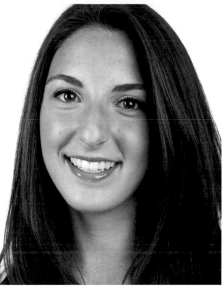

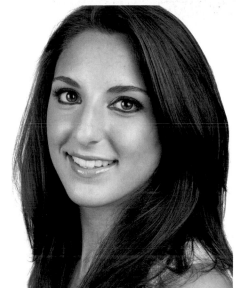

BEFORE

NATURAL LOOK

DRAMATIC LOOK

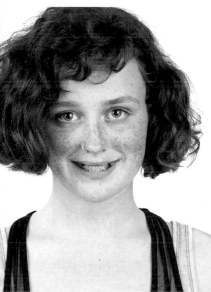

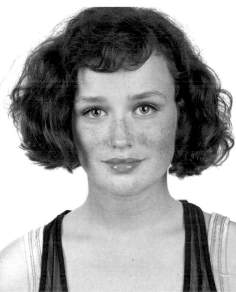

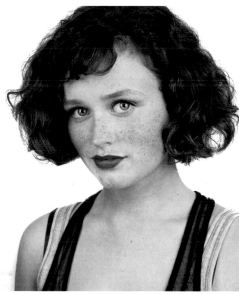

BEFORE

NATURAL LOOK

DRAMATIC LOOK

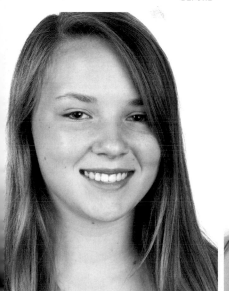

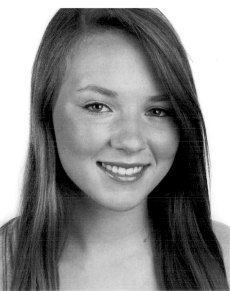

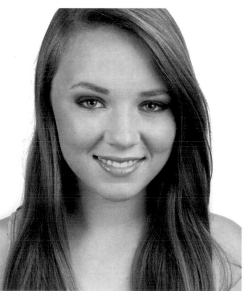

BEFORE

NATURAL LOOK

DRAMATIC LOOK

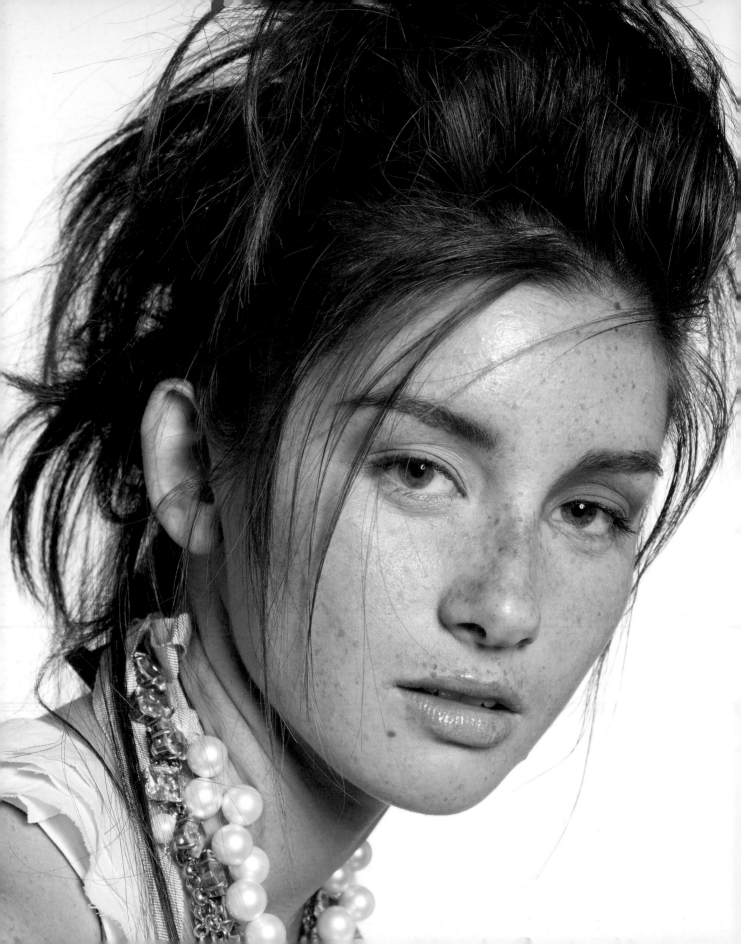

15

BEAUTY STYLE

Finding your style doesn't have to be boring. It's fun to experiment with styles for different occasions and different moods. You don't always feel the same, so why should you always look the same? Sometimes you might want to go a little edgier, sometimes preppy or sporty. If you have an interview for a job or internship, you'll need a professional appearance. For a black-tie affair, you'll want to be glamorous but appropriate. Here's how to have it all.

preppy

Preppy is collegiate, outdoorsy, and healthy. Think J. Crew, Ralph Lauren, Tory Burch, Tommy Hilfiger, Izod, Lilly Pulitzer—need I say more? So your makeup will be light. Preppy girls wear makeup, but they are so good at making you believe they aren't. You will first spend some time covering up any blemishes because preppy girls have flawless skin. Then follow with a natural blush like you just pinched your cheeks. Almost invisible eyeliner on the top only for this look. Just apply a couple coats of mascara, and then brush up your eyebrows for a super-groomed appearance. Choose a lipstick, gloss, or lip balm (the formula doesn't matter) in a color that looks like you just bit your lip. Or go Palm Beach with a bit of frosty pink.

It used to be that all preppy girls had very straight hair (or at least wanted that). Now preppy can be any kind of hair texture. You don't want to look like you had your hair set or blow-dried. You want to be neat but look like you just stepped out of bed. Headbands, either thin grosgrain or thick tortoiseshell, are great accessories.

sporty

Every athlete has her own unique style. Venus and Serena Williams love to wear rock jewelry, cool hairstyles, and even makeup on the courts. No matter what your athletic look is, you will want to stick to waterproof formulas for all your beauty products. You have to consider sweat, which will make regular mascara run (and you don't want that stuff smearing and getting in your eyes when you're trying to compete or have fun). I once saw Morgan Pressel on HDTV crying tears of joy after winning a tournament. Her black eyeliner and mascara made it through the tears! Thanks, black gel liner! Make sure when you are outside that you have adequate SPF protection either in a tinted moisturizer or underneath any makeup. Your lips should be clear, and you only need mascara on your eyes. You can also skip blush because your cheeks will be naturally flushed.

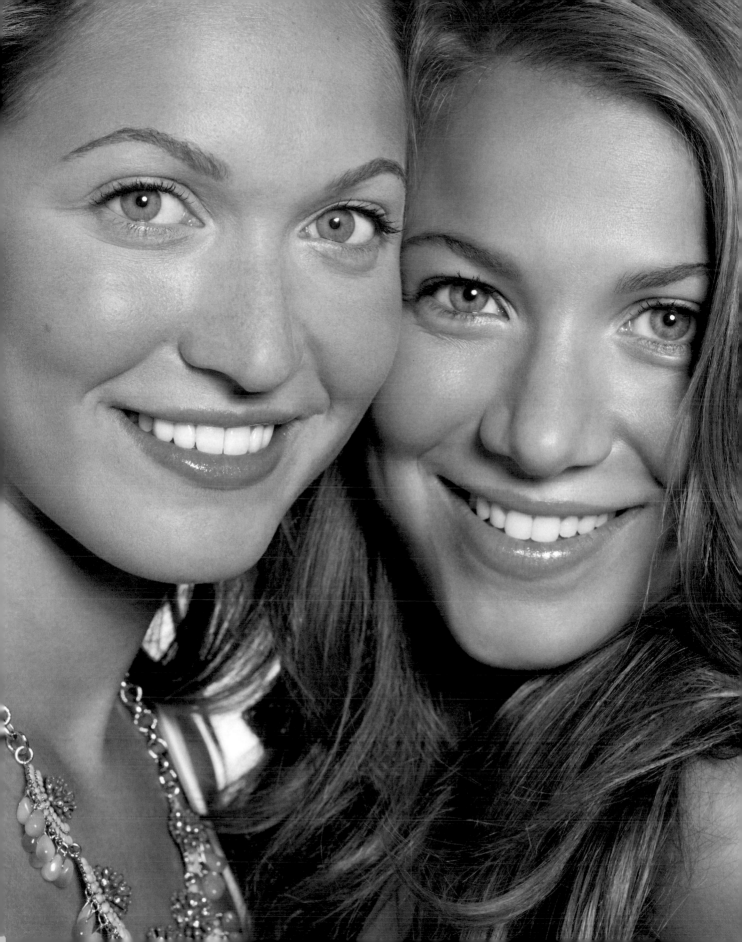

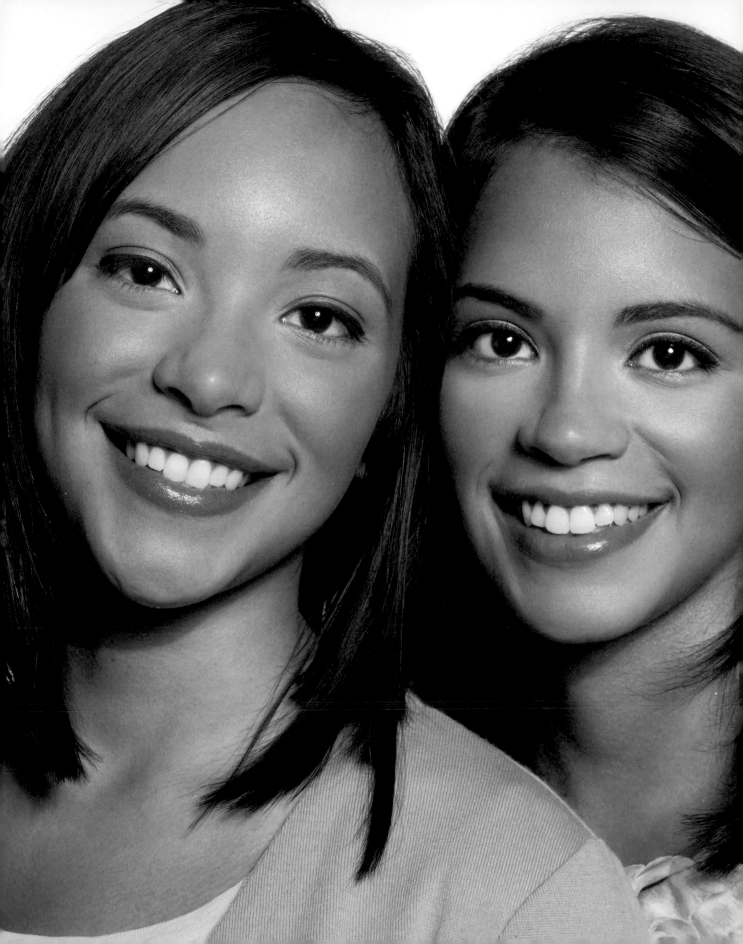

polished professional

When you have a job interview, you always want to be polished, presentable, put together, and pretty. This means your makeup should be classic, but you will most likely need concealer. I haven't met a person who doesn't look more polished with concealer under the eyes. Apply the concealer, and then even out the rest of your skin using your normal routine.

For your eyes, stick to the basics. Apply a dark brown or navy liner to the top and bottom, as well as eye shadow in a taupe or sandy shade. Curl your lashes and apply mascara. Fill in your brows very softly, and apply a bit of natural-looking blush. A touch of tinted lip balm or natural lip color is best. Pay attention to your hands, your nails should be short and impeccably groomed. Warning: under no circumstances should you have chipped nail polish (and no red or black nail polish either, please).

The clothes you wear will depend on the job you are going for. If you are headed to the White House as an intern, your look should be totally conservative (minimal jewelry, super-neat hair, pants or a skirt, a blouse, and a handbag that can hold a folder). If you are going to *Vogue,* you better look really fashionable, put together, and of the moment. No matter where you are headed, don't forget about your shoes. I notice an applicant's face first, and then I notice the shoes. Don't wear ratty old shoes, platforms, or sneakers. No sandals or flip-flops, even if it's 100 degrees outside. I love clogs, but they are not for an interview.

Another rule no matter what job you want: look people in the eye. When I meet a girl who is hunched over and looking down, I figure she isn't comfortable and confident. That makes me think the person won't be strong enough to tackle a job. Even if your stomach is doing somersaults (everyone's usually is during an interview), keep your shoulders back and your head up. Then no one will know how nervous you really are.

college party or club

When you head out to a party or club, the important thing to remember is that your makeup and outfit need to balance each other. If you are wearing something out there, keep your makeup soft. If you are going to do a strong, smoky eye, go easy with the cleavage and your skirt length.

Even if you decide to do a smoky eye, you want your makeup to look like you aren't trying too hard. You aren't on the runway or in a Gucci ad. For the perfect smoky eye, clean off the lid with face powder. Use a light color that's close to the natural shade of your lid. Start with a gray shadow with a bit of shimmer on your lid. As you move closer to the lash line apply a deeper slate-gray shadow that's matte. Closest to the lash line, use an ashy black shadow also in matte. For your liner, use a wet-looking gel liner in super-black. Add tons of black mascara. Keep your lips very subdued in a neutral color. Smoky eyes and strong lips are never paired together except for a photo shoot. Apply a bit of blush so you don't look tired. (Remember: if you're using powder shadow, do your eyes and concealer first, and clean up any messes with a non-oily makeup remover and cotton swabs before you move on to the rest of your face.)

Throw on a simple top and jeans; it really doesn't matter. Your makeup job will be so amazing, no one is going to be looking at your clothes.

edgy

The way to get this look is to experiment with trendy colors, such as ashy silver or purple metallic with silver in it for the lips. Unusual shades don't look good on everyone, so you really need to judge if they work on you.

Edgy means different, funky, and experimental. It's almost plain old ugly. But worn with confidence, it can also be kind of cool and pretty. Think Chloë Sevigny. Edgy definitely needs black liner, even for the day. The more eyeliner you put on, the stronger it looks. You can decide, depending on your normal style and comfort level, just how edgy you want to go. A little edgy—apply a medium line on the top of the eye. Super-edgy—go for lots of liner on the top and bottom of your eye (but remember, the top should always be thicker). The eyeliner should be accurately applied. Messy takes it to a place I'm not a fan of. Edgy or funky is fine as long as everything is pretty. That's the secret. Follow your black liner with a couple of coats of mascara in black. To soften all the gray and black on your face, add a little blush in your natural tone.

This style definitely doesn't work with a scowl. I like the edgy look best for girls who smile and get good grades. It's an unexpected twist for the good girl.

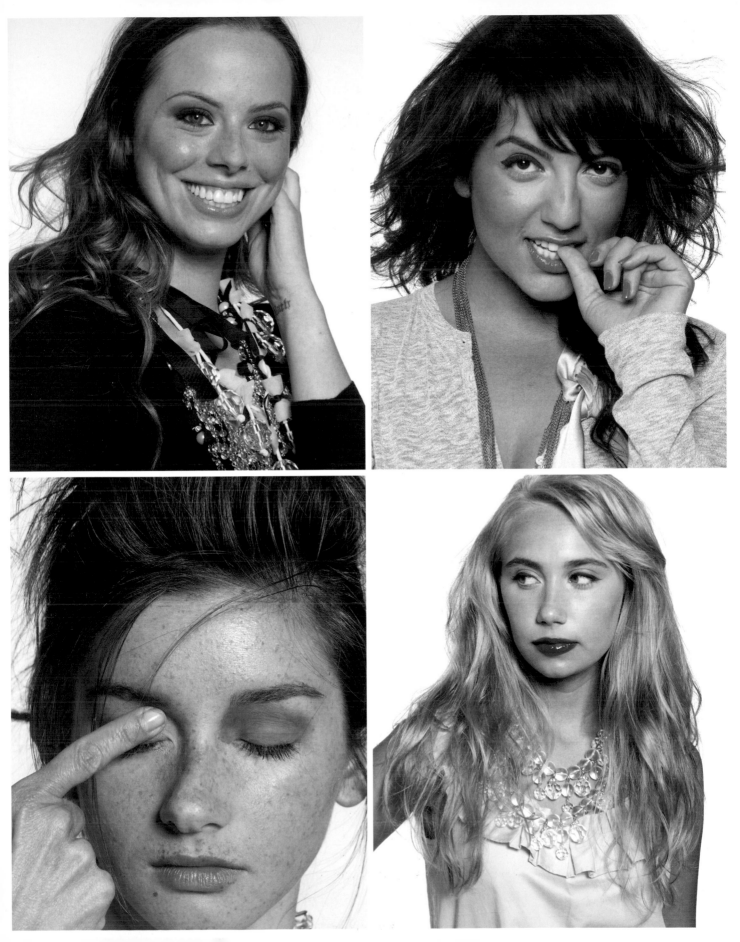

romantic

You don't need a lot of makeup for a romantic look. Your skin should be very peaches and cream, which you can achieve by first evening out your skin tone with whatever foundation, tinted moisturizer, or makeup stick you use. Then make your cheeks look extra flushed by picking a color that's in the pastel pink family (deeper plum works on darker skin). You don't want to use your normal blush, which matches the color of your cheeks when you are exercising, because working out is great but definitely not romantic. Use a little bit more of the soft, pastel color on the apples of the cheeks than you normally use. Because the color is pretty fair, don't worry about using more than usual. Make sure it is well blended so it almost looks like you have been embarrassed.

Create romantic rosebud lips by choosing a tinted lip balm in a pinkish, half-shade-softer tone than your natural color. For darker lips, go for rose tones. They will give the same look. The effect will be sweet with a little sheen. Your eyes should complement the understated and soft tones in your face. Use some soft smudged shadow in a natural brown color just above the lash line and then follow with brown-black mascara.

Your hair should be an ethereal border to your beautiful face. Think of Victorian hair, either pinned loosely around the face or free-flowing and soft. You can't really mess it up.

black tie

A black-tie event is not the same as walking the red carpet. Aim to be classy, not dramatic or funky. There will be a lot of grown-ups with jewelry and nice clothes. (And if you're the girlfriend, everyone will be looking at you.)

Start with a polished face, employing your regimen of concealer, foundation, and blush. Remember the rules of proportions. If you opt for a conservative dress with some pearls, go for a stronger, smoky eye. If your outfit is sexier, try a red or deep rosy lip with a bit of shimmer on the eyes and some black mascara.

Here's something I've learned from years of attending black-tie events: if you do go with that dress with the plunging neckline, make sure you bring a wrap. You might have felt great showing off your cleavage while you got dressed in the privacy of your own home. But once you show up at the event and wind up talking to Great-Aunt Milly, you might feel different. Plus, a lot of ballrooms get really cold.

My other black-tie rule of thumb: if you find yourself struggling with bra strap or underwear lines at home, change. The problem is only going to get worse once you are out. And the point of the party is to have fun. So be comfortable.

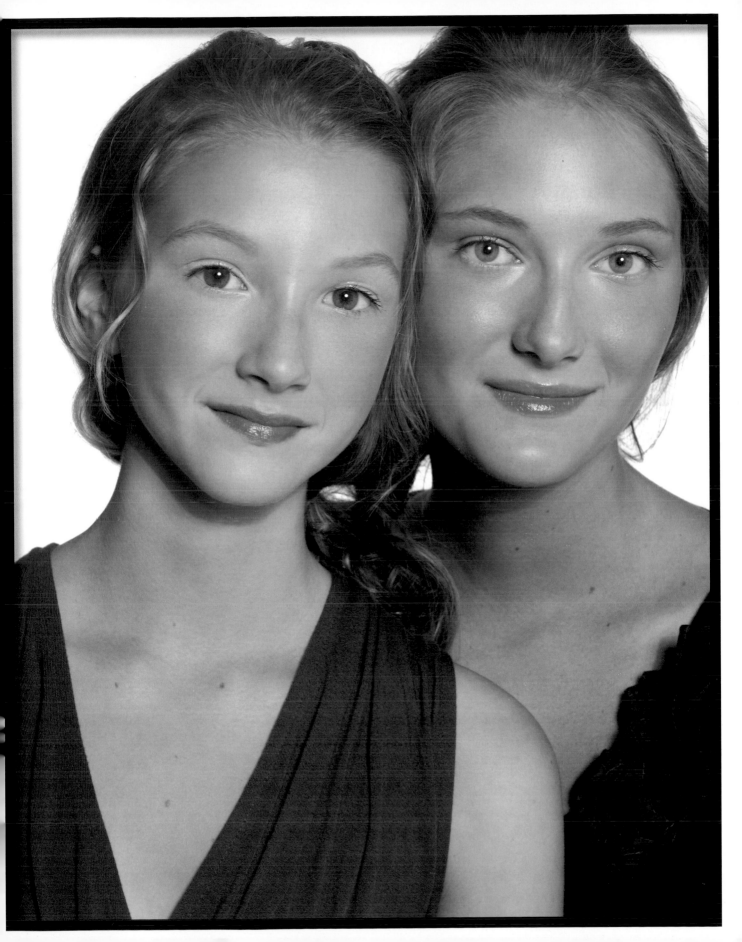

PICTURE PERFECT

Photos are everywhere. They are online, on our mobiles and cell phones, in places I never thought I would see them. You can't look great in every photo taken of you. But for the ones that count, makeup plays a big role. When I look at old photos of myself, I see that my makeup was applied heavier than I would like it now. I don't look fresh or modern at all. You don't need a lot of makeup in a picture to look good. And certainly, less makeup looks better than the wrong makeup. Concealer, bronzer, and the right blush always make you look better in photos. They smooth the skin and give you a little bit of standout quality. The other photo essentials are groomed eyebrows and mascara, which make even the most beautiful girl look better.

online photos

Your image is about much more than what your makeup looks like in a picture. It's about everything you project in a photo, from the clothes you wear to the stance you take to what you are doing.

Once you put something online, there is no taking it back. I know you know this, but even if you erase a picture from your Facebook page, it might be too late. Someone else may have taken that photo and spread it around. So be careful of what you put out there. Think about how you are presenting yourself. I'm not a fan of girls who plaster their pages with photos of themselves with black-rimmed eyes and hair swept to the side and doing provocative poses. This kind of thing might seem funny when your boyfriend or friends snap a shot with their phone at a party or club. But when you don't get a job because a potential employer checks out your Facebook page (we all do), it's not as funny. Everything you do—from your screen name to your online page—tells someone who you are. Protect and respect your image.

yearbook

Here's the main thing with yearbook photos: don't ever expect them to look good. They all look the same—kind of goofy, sort of sweet, definitely age appropriate. If you look fine, be happy. They are timeless and funny. Make sure you get one, even if it scares you to look at it. You need to give your kids something to chuckle at in the future.

retouched photos

We are all so screwed up when it comes to how we look in photos because of the widespread use of retouching in commercial and editorial pictures. Pretty much every single professional photo you see, whether it's in a book, magazine, or ad campaign, has been altered in Photoshop after it's been shot. The trick is to make the retouched photos look like they're not retouched. But if you compare closely the same celebrity on different magazine covers, you will see different body shapes, eye color, noses, even smiles. The computer-generated changes of most photos are hard for the untrained eye to detect. But the overall effect is that we have an unrealistic expectation of how we should look, in photos and real life. Know this as you are judging unretouched photos of yourself, and be kind to your real beauty.

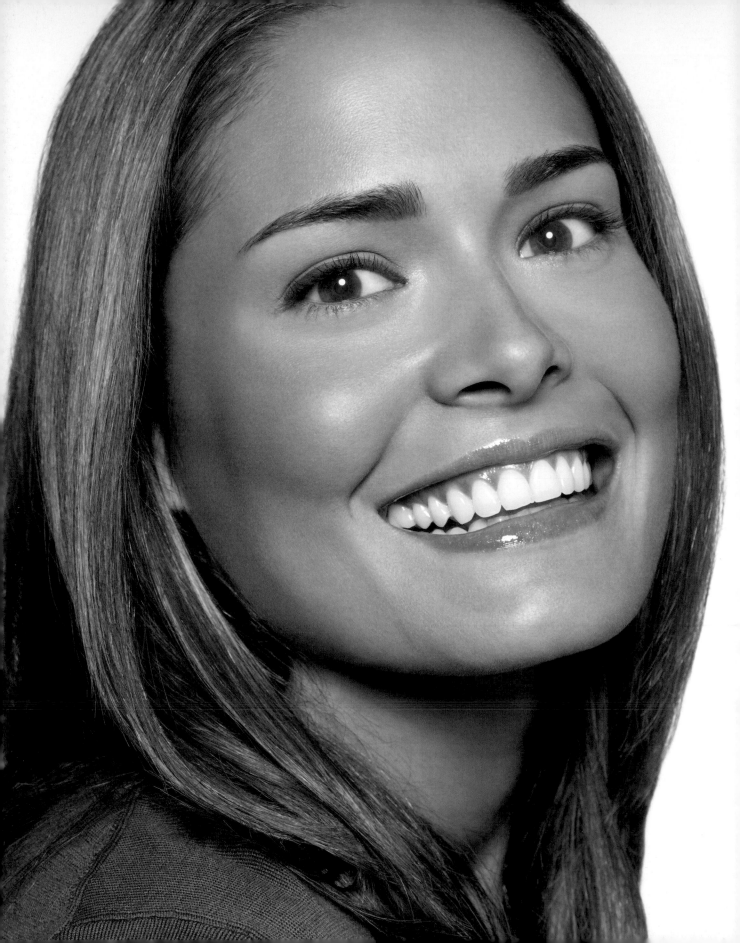

16

MODEL LIFE

I meet so many girls who want to be models. It doesn't matter if they are 6 feet tall or 5 feet tall. Blond or brunette. Waifs or glamazons. Modeling appears to be very glamorous and exciting. That is partly true. But it's also a very tough business.

I have been working with models ever since the day I started in the industry. Just like with any other job, there are nice people and not-so-nice ones. It's been cool to work with the most beautiful, famous, and interesting models in the world since they were teens (I began working with Naomi Campbell when she was fourteen and Niki Taylor when she was only thirteen). But it doesn't matter how pretty someone is; models have insecurities, too.

The truth is, many girls I see on the street in my town are a lot prettier than the professional models I work with. That's because modeling isn't just about being pretty. It's about having a certain look and photographing well. To make it in the business, you generally have to be really tall (over 5 feet 10 inches), be überskinny (that means not a lot of muscle), and have the look (it used to be Barbie Doll, and now it's more unusual and androgynous).

Classic beauty, which might make a girl popular at school, isn't always what the modeling industry is looking for.

Modeling is not pure glamour. There are good parts and bad parts. If you are successful, you travel all over the world, make good money, and meet interesting people. But every day of your life, someone gets to say whether you are amazing or awful. If you look tired, gained a few pounds, or just don't have the right look, you will hear about it. The judgment is not based on how well you play the piano, or that you got an A on your report, or the incredible goal you scored at your match. You are judged solely on your looks. There's nothing pretty about that.

model behavior

Maybe you really do want to be a model, or people have told you that you should be one and you are curious. There's nothing wrong with giving it a try, but you need to educate yourself. Here's important advice on being smart about the biz.

DOs

DO get permission from your family. Modeling is a group effort so you will need their support and counsel. Keep them in the loop on all decisions, and listen if they tell you something isn't a good idea. They are probably right.

DO have a friend who is good at photography take photos to send to agencies. You don't need to pay money to hire a professional photographer. Find a friend who's good with a camera to snap simple shots. Agencies can tell if they are interested right away and aren't impressed with fancy lighting or angles. Keep your hair and makeup simple! Agents want to see you. Send a full-length picture and a headshot.

DO look neat, simple, and comfortable if you get called in by an agency for a "go see." Arrive in simple clothes like jeans, T-shirts, and sneakers, with little makeup.

DO let it go if it isn't working. There are lots of reasons why modeling might not be the right fit for you. Maybe you don't have the look agencies are interested in right now. Or you don't like the atmosphere on photo shoots. If it's not right, channel your initial interest in the profession into something else, like an acting class, commercials, makeup, or styling.

DON'Ts

DON'T sign up for modeling school. Modeling schools only benefit the people collecting the tuition fees. Anything you learn about modeling will happen on the job through listening to and watching photographers, stylists, makeup artists, and other models.

DON'T go local. Unless you happen to live in New York City, Miami, Los Angeles, or London. If you live in a small town, skip your local modeling agencies and write to agencies in those cities, where the modeling industry resides.

DON'T give up if one agency rejects you. If an agent deems you unfit for modeling, move on and try two or three other agencies. Everyone sees something different.

DON'T pay money to an agency that signs you. You shouldn't have to fork over a single penny if the agency is reputable. If an agent asks you to pay for a test photo session, hair and makeup for the session, or assembling a portfolio, move on.

DON'T starve yourself to become an unnatural body type. There is a lot of pressure in the modeling world to be thin, but if you stop eating to please an agent or photographer, you are putting yourself in danger. Talk to your parents, a friend who is not in the business, or your doctor if you are obsessing over food. (Read *Hungry: A Young Model's Story of Appetite, Ambition, and the Ultimate Embrace of Curves,* a book by now-plus-size model Crystal Renn about her struggle to stay unnaturally thin.)

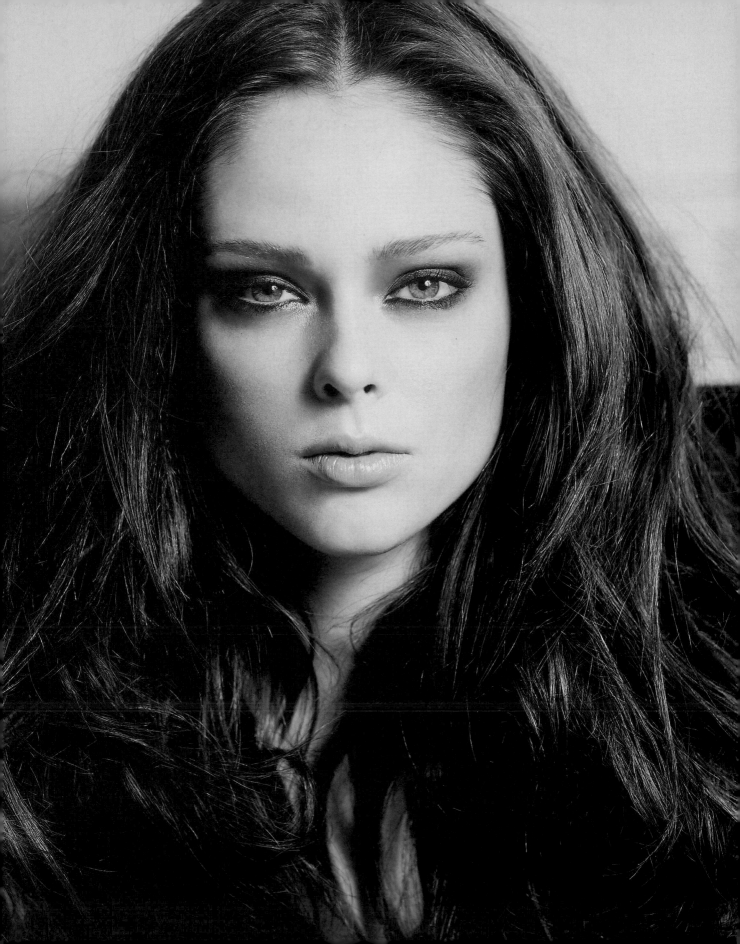

INTERVIEW: COCO ROCHA
A MODEL ON A MISSION

This twenty-year-old Canadian is a rare breed. Coco has made it as a high-fashion model, gracing the hottest runways and most important magazines in the world. But she hasn't sacrificed her beliefs for the sake of her career. She won't pose nude or with cigarettes. And most important, Coco is outspoken on the issue of eating disorders in her business and what the fashion industry can do to combat the problem.

How did you get your start as a model?

When I was fourteen, I was in an Irish dance competition (I had been training since I was about six years old) where an agent, who had a daughter dancing, asked me if I was interested in modeling. It was a complete surprise. I was not the pretty or popular girl in school. My friends and I were all laughing. They thought it was hopeless.

What kind of teen were you?

I was the tall, gangly girl. Dance was my life. I wasn't attractive. I didn't wear my hair in a special way or any makeup. I didn't have a stylish wardrobe. With my friends, I was outgoing. Around guys or the popular girls, I was a little nervous and taken aback. You can ask any model; she wasn't the attractive girl in school. That's my favorite part of the model's life: she wasn't the girl who was expected to go far with her looks. It's a Cinderella story.

What was it like when you first started modeling?

Runway was pretty easy for me. Photo shoots weren't enjoyable because I wasn't comfortable. I was fine with my body and my image, but I didn't find myself sexy. When you think of a model, you think beautiful, gorgeous, sexy. You don't think of a fourteen-year-old girl scared out of her mind. Taking those pictures was hard. When I started I was nervous about what people thought of me.

Was that as hard as it sounds?

Rejection makes you stronger. At first it sucks, but then you learn from it. Girls who do well learn how to take rejection without being insulted. Some people will say things that are so unbelievable. To an average person it would be so insulting, but it's our jobs. They'll say you are too big, or they don't like your face, or they don't think you are edgy enough. It comes with the paycheck. That is what you learn: it is all about image.

How did you learn to deal with all that rejection in a healthy way?

When I was sixteen, I went to Singapore and lost a lot of weight by eating healthily and working out a lot. I worked so hard at the gym that I went from 118 to 108 pounds [Coco is 5 feet 9 inches]. After all that, I had a person say to me, "The look is anorexic," and told me to lose more. I thought to myself, "I lost all this weight and still I am not good enough." I realized that they want you to get every job, but you can't. If you don't like me today, someone else is going to like me tomorrow. I'm glad I learned it early in my career. I want to stick to my morals and beliefs. Sometimes when I'm asked to do things and I say no, a lot of people say that's risky for my career. But I got to do what I got to do. I don't want to ruin my life.

How much do you weigh now?

I weigh 130 pounds. My body is a lot of muscle from dance.

A lot of girls might have had a different reaction to what happened to you. Where do you find your strength to stay true to yourself?

I have a strong mom. If I ever did something that I thought was unsafe, my mom would say, "You are done." I was brought up as a Jehovah's Witness. We have strict beliefs. I stay believing what I believe. I have had moments where I fell because of peer pressure. But now, I like being a model, who can voice a lot of things.

One of the things you are outspoken about is the issue of eating disorders in the industry. How did that happen?

The industry was talking about the issue, but nobody was asking the models. Girls needed to say what they thought because it is all about their health and their bodies. Five years from now, I have to live with my body and won't be part of the industry. I was starting to talk about it more and more. *Vogue* editor in chief Anna Wintour heard my interviews and asked me to talk about models with eating disorders at a health initiative held by the Council of Fashion Designers of America. That was a major milestone to have the backing of *Vogue*. These are lives that we are working with and not just racks.

What initiatives did you recommend the fashion industry take?

During fashion shows, they have food backstage. But they aren't the greatest foods to be eating, like cakes and pastries. I asked if they could keep out more food and a better variety. Also, for the shows, designers pick one girl to fit all the clothes on beforehand. I talked about making sure that girl is a healthy size.

Have things changed?

Things have not changed drastically, but it's much better than it was. If a lot of girls started to speak out, there would be a solution. It's a hard subject, but there are more models coming out and talking about it, which is exciting to see.

What's your advice to girls who want to get into the business?

Keep true to yourself. This job doesn't last that long. The average modeling career is about five years. You need to make sure that you are OK and doing fine, because you need to walk out of this and say I'm still me and still good.

Why do people idolize models so much?

They look at our pictures, and think, "I want to be that girl on the cover of that magazine." I look at that same picture of myself and think the same thing. They don't realize everything that goes into that picture—the hours of makeup, hair, and styling; the editing of the pictures; and the retouching. Girls need to step back and say that is not the exact replica.

What's the best part of your job?

You get to travel, meet people, learn a life that most will never experience, just being around people who are the most influential people in the world—and at only sixteen years old!

Any other perks?

We learn how to wear makeup and get to keep a lot of it. I am a makeup fanatic. I'm very pale, so when I don't wear makeup, I look very sick. I am so white with freckles. I need a little bit of shading and color. I have tons of makeup. One section of my closet is just makeup. One of my favorite products is Bobbi Brown's BBU Palette, which is a huge palette with foundation for every skin color.

What do you do on your off time?

I love to listen to music and read books. When I'm back in Vancouver, I hang out with friends and have sleepovers. I don't go to crazy parties. I will go to some events to show my support for designers and editors. But if it's just about me, I go to movies and hang out with friends. I'm the Average Joe girl.

INTERVIEW: MANDA GARCIA
THE MODEL WITH IT ALL

This thirty-three-year-old New Jersey native has been working ever since I discovered her in a local pizzeria when she was thirteen years old. Now a mom of two boys, Manda juggles work and life with true beauty (see her beautiful photo on page 238).

How did you get your start as a model?

Bobbi was picking up pizza and saw me and asked if I was interested in modeling. I was only in eighth grade and was pretty shy. She gave me a phone number, but I didn't call. So when she saw me a couple of weeks later, Bobbi set up some appointments for me to go to agencies. I picked one and that is how I got started. . . . When I was twenty-four years old, I had a casting for Bobbi's line. I happened to see her when we were in the waiting room. I showed her my book, and then I said, "You don't remember me." She looked at me with a strange look. I told her the story and it all came back to her. Then I ended up doing the ad campaign!

What was your career like when you were a teen?

My first job was working for *Seventeen* magazine. I remember being the youngest person on the shoot for a long time. . . . In high school, I worked throughout the year. I had to go on castings and appointments. I was able to work as long as I kept my schoolwork up.

How did you manage modeling with your schoolwork?

I made sure I didn't overload myself. If I felt like it was too much, I would decline the job and say I can't do it right now. The teachers and principal worked with me. I did my work on the side. I had to study. Even though modeling is fun, it is still work. You had to balance all these things. School is the most important thing.

It sounds like you had a normal life.

Modeling was just a job for me. I didn't want to make it my life. I wanted to have other aspects to my life, like having fun, getting pizza, and going to the mall. I'm happy I didn't give that up. I lived in Paris for a year after high school. There were girls there who were younger and had dropped out of school. I was happy I didn't do that. You can be too young to be on your own in a different country.

What do you love about being a model?

I always loved the process of going through makeup and hair and having a stylist. You don't have input on what is going on. I like how you don't have much control. The product that comes out is cool. It's a crunch of ideas that get thrown together. You have a certain style, so it is nice to see someone else's idea of how you can look.

What was one of your best experiences as a model?

I remember going to Greece when I was twenty-six to do a shoot of wedding gowns. That was really beautiful. It was really picturesque. I could bring my mom, and it was a weeklong shoot, so we were able to see a lot of Greece.

What kind of makeup do you wear in real life?

I like very natural, easygoing makeup. I do like to put on some makeup if I am going out—a little concealer, mascara, powder, blush, and lip gloss. Just enough so that it seems like you look great naturally.

What's your exercise routine?

I have always been a runner. I try to do a lot of working out outside. It makes me feel better. I will try anything once. I have done kickboxing. I try to give everything a chance.

How about your diet?

I like to eat really healthily. I can never follow a strict diet. I focus on eating lots of fruits and veggies and whole grains and cheeses. I am not a vegetarian, but I could be. I don't really do any sort of limiting. If I want a little piece of chocolate, I'll have it. Everything in moderation.

You've been a model for almost twenty years. That's a long time!

It used to be that when you were twenty-three, you were almost done with your career. Now there is a lot more work. I never thought I would still be working at this point. Now it is better than ever.

What advice do you have for girls who want to get into the business?

Try and go for it. Don't let anyone make you feel like you can't do something.

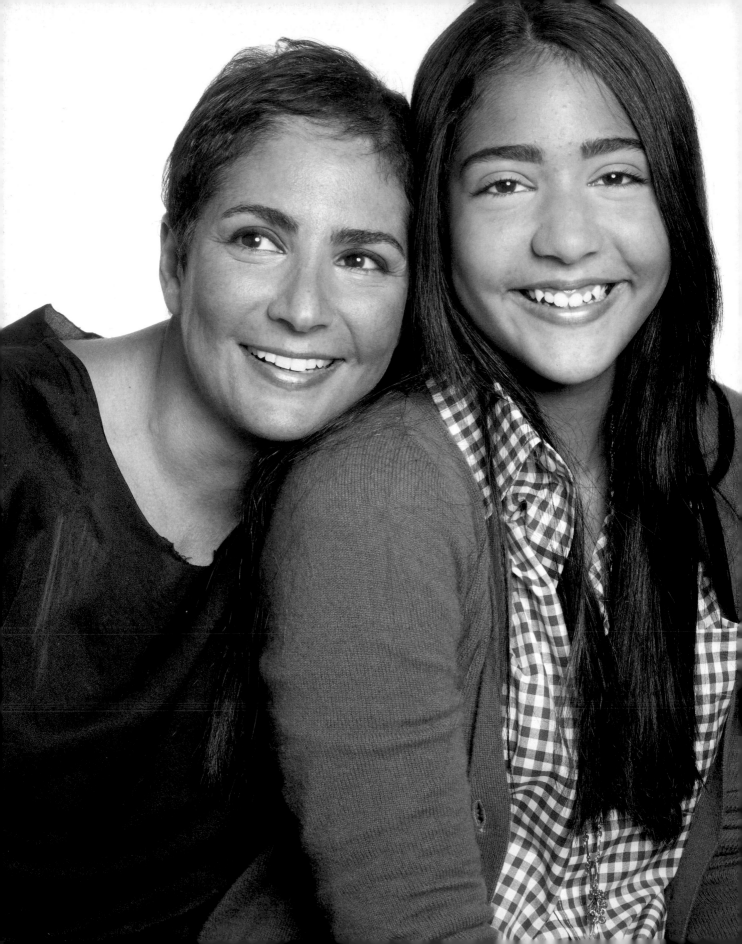

17

MOMS AND DAUGHTERS

Dear Moms,
Mothers and daughters have this incredible love. Sometimes it is difficult for moms to separate from their daughters and realize that there are two individual people here. As a mom, you want to see your kids succeed so badly you'll do anything, even relive your own childhood traumas. If you were teased for your weight as a kid, you might worry about your daughter going through the same thing and try to prevent it. But everyone has her own destiny.

I remember once when I was doing a makeup demonstration for a group of Girl Scouts, one of the mothers stood up during the question-answer period and began talking about her daughter's bad eating habits. While this woman went on and on, her daughter sunk deeper and deeper into her chair. I understand where the mom was coming from—she only wanted the best for her daughter—but by pointing out her kid's flaws in public, she wound up hurting her.

Don't point out your daughter's flaws. Instead, help her embrace who she is. I know you might be worried that your daughter is a couple of pounds heavier than you think she should be. Or maybe she's decided to dye her beautiful blond hair jet black, much to your horror. Girls need to go through certain experiences, and you need to let them. It's important to lead and teach your daughter, but then hang back and give her a little space. Keep your insecurities about yourself to yourself as much as you can (that's what your friends are for).

The biggest gifts a mom can give a daughter are self-love and self-confidence. My mother always told me I was beautiful and wonderful and talented and smart when I was a young kid. It gave me the confidence to go on and do what I do in life. One of my greatest talents is being naive to the idea that there isn't anything I can't do. That's thanks to my mother.

Give that to your daughter through action and words. Encourage your daughter to play sports by showing up at her games. In fact, show an interest in anything she does. If your daughter struggles with something, find a way to make it more positive. That can mean going to a yoga or spinning class together if she's resistant to exercising. Try planning and cooking dinner together if you are worried about her nutrition. If she's uncomfortable about her style, go through her closet with her to sort out what should be tailored or tossed. Do fun beauty things together like getting your nails done or hitting the makeup counter. Don't forget to tell your daughter she is beautiful, smart, and, most important, that you love her.

Dear Daughters,

Your mother loves you. You have to know that, no matter what happens. And you have to understand the reason she is doing all those things that upset you—punishing you because you didn't do your homework, telling you to stand up straight, making you sit down for dinner with the family—is because that's her job.

Believe it or not, your mother was once your age. All mothers were once teenagers and probably didn't feel that differently than you do now. One day—it might be when you are in your twenties or after you become a mom yourself—it will hit you that your mom has always been on your side. You'll realize and appreciate all the sacrifices she made for you, like staying up all night with you as a baby or wearing the same clothes so you can buy a new wardrobe every season. It's a part of the process.

Until then, try to see your mom as more than, well, just a mom. I love looking at pictures of my mom when she was young. I asked her lots of questions about her life, like how did she feel going to the prom or know my dad was the one for her. Get to know your mom from different times of her life.

Listen to your mom when she gives you important life rules, like wearing your seatbelt, not smoking, and letting her know where you are after school and at night. Understand the difference between that kind of stuff and the negotiable rules. If your mom doesn't think black eyeliner is appropriate, OK, go for a dark brown. Not such a big deal.

Communication is everything in all relationships but especially with your mom. Don't be afraid to tell her your problems and things that you need. No matter how hard it is, I promise you that it will get better. For right now, all you have to do is just say thanks for being a good mother. It goes a long way.

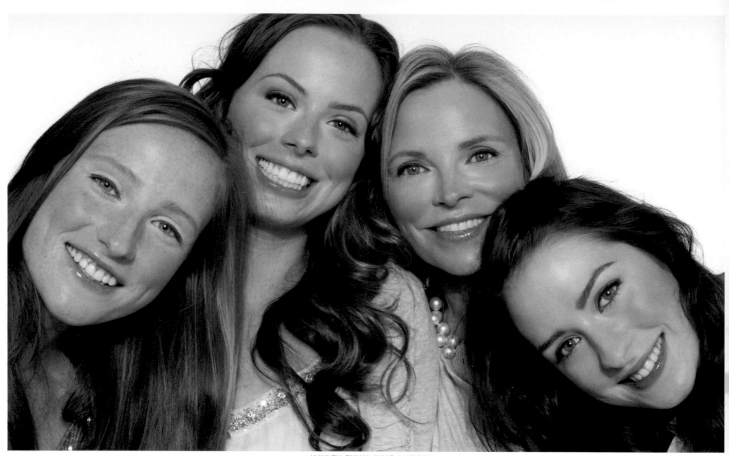

HAYLEY, EMILY, JULIE, LINDSEY

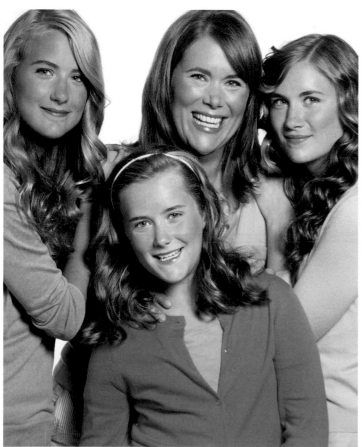

KAILA, MAGGIE, MELISSA, SAVANNAH

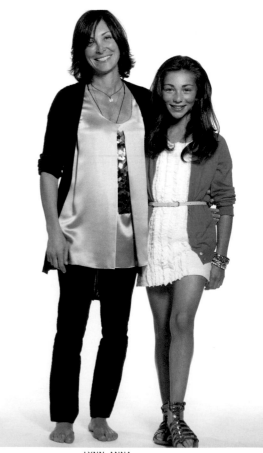

LYNN, ANNA

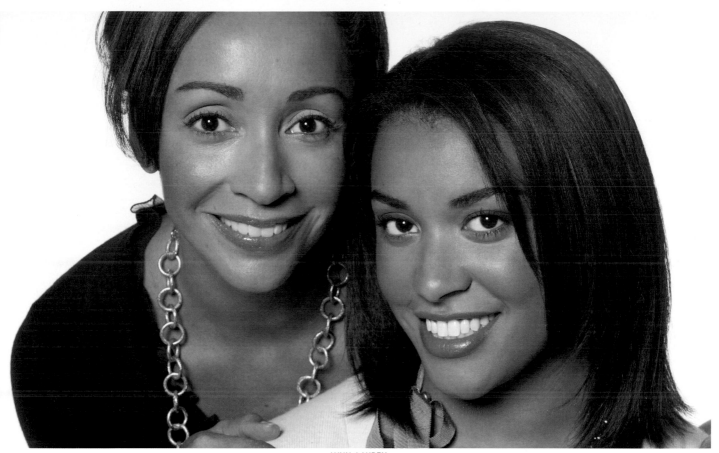

LYNN, LAUREN

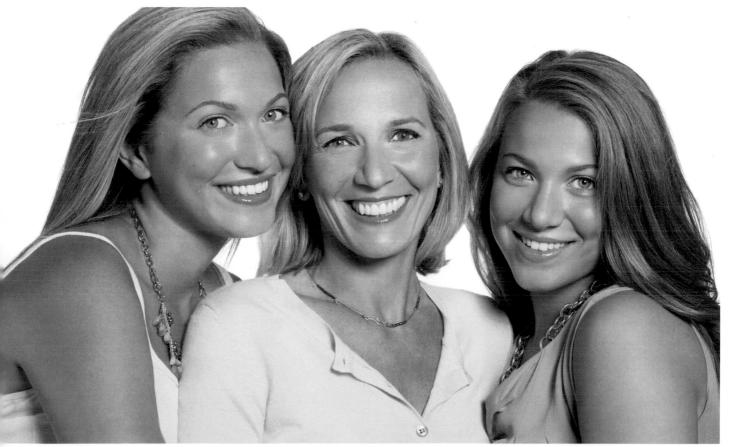

MARGARET, JILL, ELIZABETH

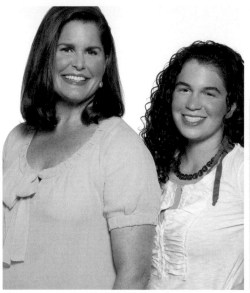

ALEXANDRA, GRACE

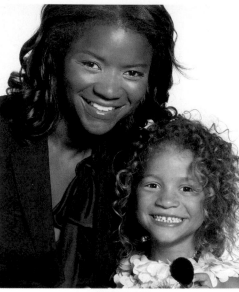

JACQUIE, REMI

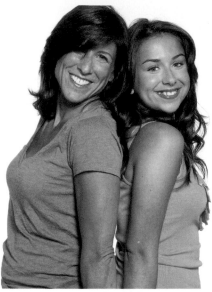

LAINIE, SAMANTHA

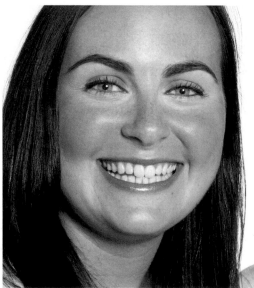

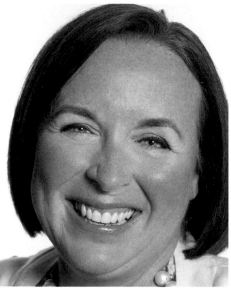

KELSEY, DARA

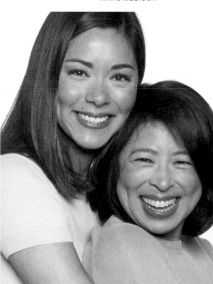

MIMI, MELISSA

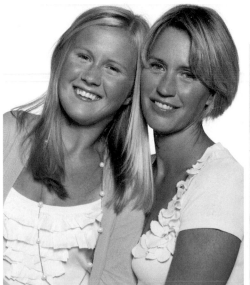

WHITNEY, HILLARY

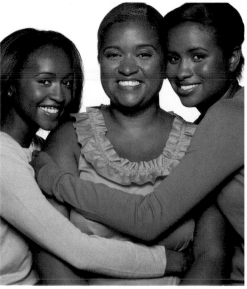

JAYANNA, MARIAELENA, MARLENNE

AMANDA, ALICE

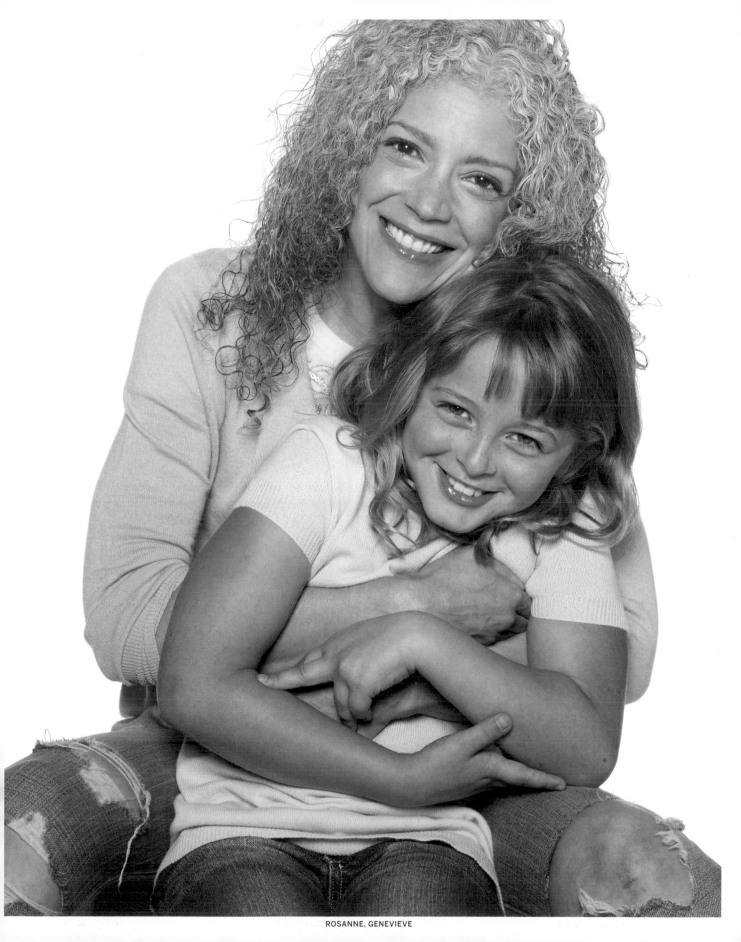

ROSANNE, GENEVIEVE

MODEL MOMS

There's often a lot of expectation that daughters will be like their moms. This can put pressure on all kinds of girls, but can you imagine if your mom were a famous model?

The comparisons seem like they would be brutal.

These moms and daughters have handled their relationships beautifully...

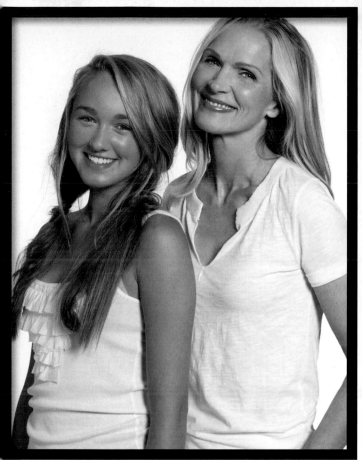

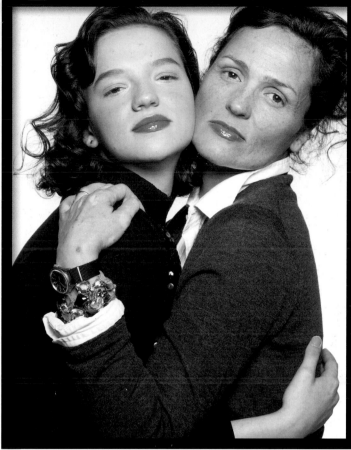

MOM: DIANNE

Adrienne has heard—and seen in the celebrity and model worlds—that exotic, unusual, or out-of-the-ordinary beauty is quite compelling. Beauty-pageant beauty is far from the only kind of beautiful. Adrienne and I comment on a person's attractive smile, an unusual nose, special eyes, or outstanding hair. We also find that the way someone behaves or how they speak makes the whole package of beautiful. Many models photographed have a beauty all their own, not cookie-cutter or overly gorgeous. I hope that Adrienne sees her own beauty.

DAUGHTER: ADRIENNE

I love going through my mom's closet. All of her clothes are beautiful, and because she was gifted with so much expensive designer clothing, we are very careful about our purchases and buy most everything on sale! My favorite tip from her is to wear an oversize sweater for comfort, and it will always look stylish with a cute belt. She also always says that whenever something may go out of style, it almost always comes back "in" again. . . . I find it the greatest compliment when people say that I look like her. She is beautiful, and I'm very glad I got some of her amazing genes.

MOM: MARISA

For me, staying in the physical condition that modeling required was a high price to pay. I was never naturally skinny. I wasted so much of my time thinking about not eating rather than just living. I never wanted this for my daughter. I shared my experiences with her so that she could see the whole picture, rather than just the things we see in the media. I wanted her to understand the cost of that kind of career, and understand the importance of balance—beauty is emotional, physical, and spiritual.

DAUGHTER: JUSTINE

My mom is my mentor. She gives me the courage to carry out my ideas, including creating my clothing line, Academy for Wayward Girls. She takes me to shoots and shows so I can learn how things work. She also loves to photograph me and reminds me that what makes me different are the things that give me a special beauty.

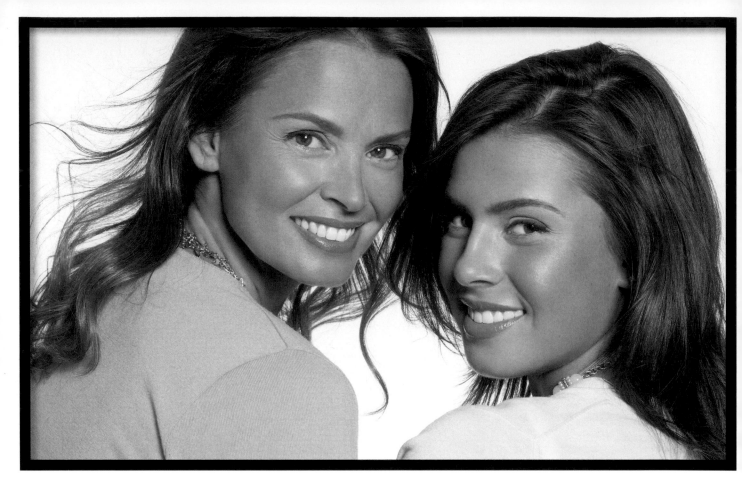

MOM: KARINA

I admire my daughter immensely. Marielle is the girl I would have been in awe of if we were in high school together. She is confident, beautiful, athletic, loyal, artistic, smart, and funny. I've always told her that and remind her all the time. . . . I never focused too much on being a model. I am a mother, wife, daughter, sister, and friend first. Everything else follows.

DAUGHTER: MARIELLE

Early on, I thought that I was going to be a model like my mom. Her job looked like so much fun. I told myself that when I was 16, I was going to try out modeling. But as I grew up, reality kicked in. A model has to be tall and really skinny. My athletic build and height of 5 feet 7 inches didn't quite make the cut. I'm not bothered by the fact that I can't be a model because I'm happy with the way I look. My mom gives me confidence in every aspect of my life. Getting a compliment from someone who's in the "beauty business" is the ultimate ego-booster.

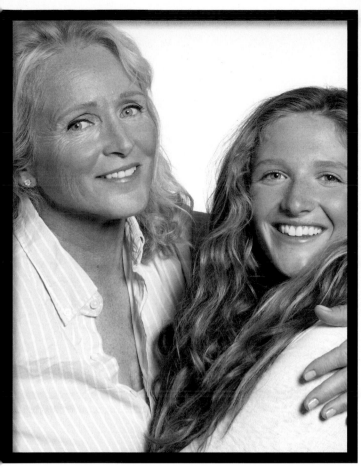

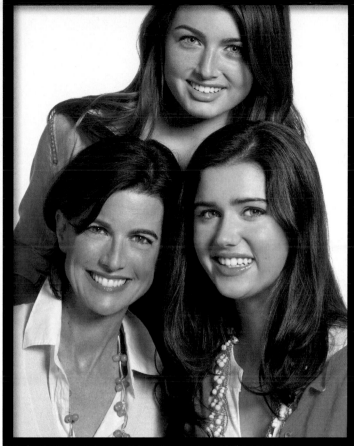

MOM: JANE

I have always made it a point to tell Grace about how much airbrushing and Photoshopping goes on with a photo of someone in a magazine. Girls today can lose so much confidence if they feel like they will never look like that girl in the magazine. It's so important that girls know the truth. . . . Through modeling, I have lifelong friends, who have become important to Grace. Bruce Weber [famed fashion photographer] is her godfather. *Vogue*'s creative director, Grace Coddington, always gives her cool things that she may have from the *Vogue* closet.

DAUGHTER: GRACE

My mom has an awesome sense of style. She's been teaching me ever since I was young not always to go for the big brand names and to look for the funky stuff. It's fun, and most of the time I'm not wearing the same thing as someone else. . . . People have expectations that I will be super-photogenic, so even with candid shots I try and look my best.

MOM: MARY (WITH DAUGHTERS MOLLY AND REILLY)

I'm a very honest mom with my girls and have always told them, when asked, if I didn't think their outfit or makeup was working . . . but I have always told them every day of their lives how beautiful I think they are, inside and out.

DAUGHTER: REILLY

There are some days where, unfortunately, even at forty-nine she looks better than I do at sixteen. She's shared countless amazing recommendations for makeup and maintaining inner and outer beauty (mostly inner). She's also stressed the importance of never having chipped nail polish or over-plucking your eyebrows. . . . She's definitely a role model, best friend, and mother. She's taught me that beauty comes with confidence in yourself, even on the off days we all have.

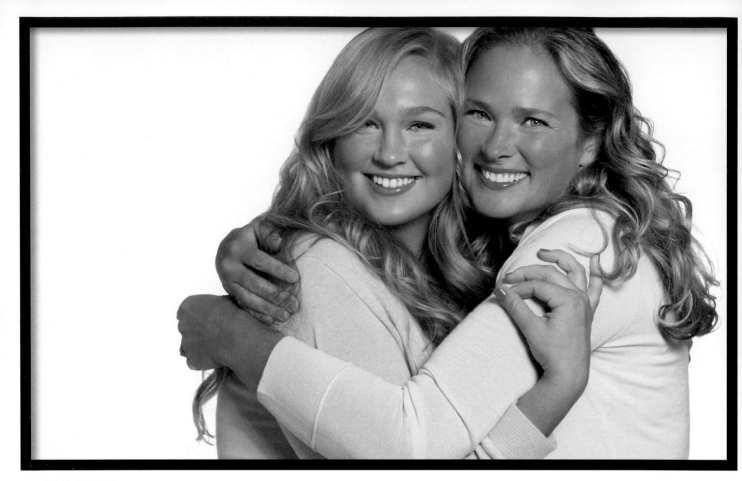

MOM: NANCY

If it wasn't hard enough growing up with a mom who was a model, Genevieve's dad is also a fashion photographer. My daughter is a beautiful girl, and might have been able to model, but our way of protecting her from any kind of rejection from a pretty superficial industry was to tell her if she wanted to try it, she had to wait until she was sixteen. Mind you, there are great folks out there—Bobbi is one of them—but it can be tough. Fortunately, she had no interest in modeling, so that was never an issue. I think we both have weight issues, mentally and physically, and I wish it wasn't the case. Think of all of the brain cells we waste on wondering if we look fat in something!

DAUGHTER: GENEVIEVE

My siblings and I weren't brought up in the way that my mom's modeling is a huge part of our lives. She isn't hung up about it. She's just taught me how to be honest and good to people.

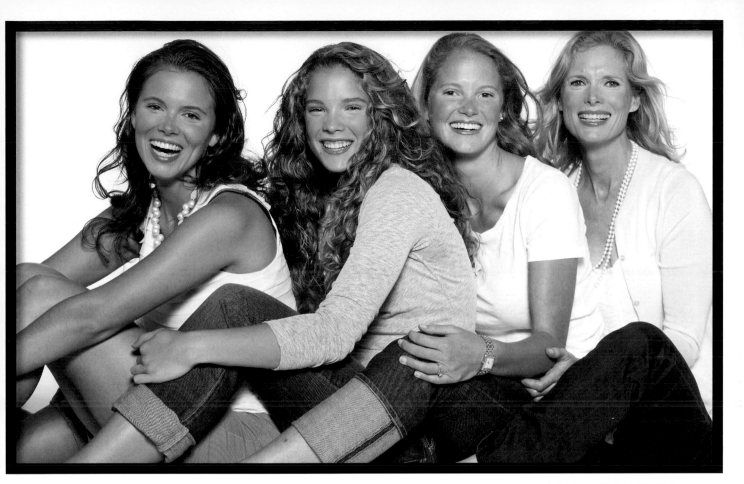

MOM: LISA (WITH DAUGHTERS STEPHANIE, ALEXIS, AND KELLY)

I tried not to put too much emphasis on external beauty, although I would always tell my daughters when they looked particularly lovely. I think my comments are more about one aspect, like "Your hair looks really great today" or "You look really great in that outfit." rather than "You are so beautiful."

DAUGHTER: KELLY

It's pretty cool to have a mom who's in with the modeling business. I think many kids are jealous when I tell them I'm going to do this or that, something they could only dream about doing. It's fun to hear all her stories about modeling and it makes me want to model.

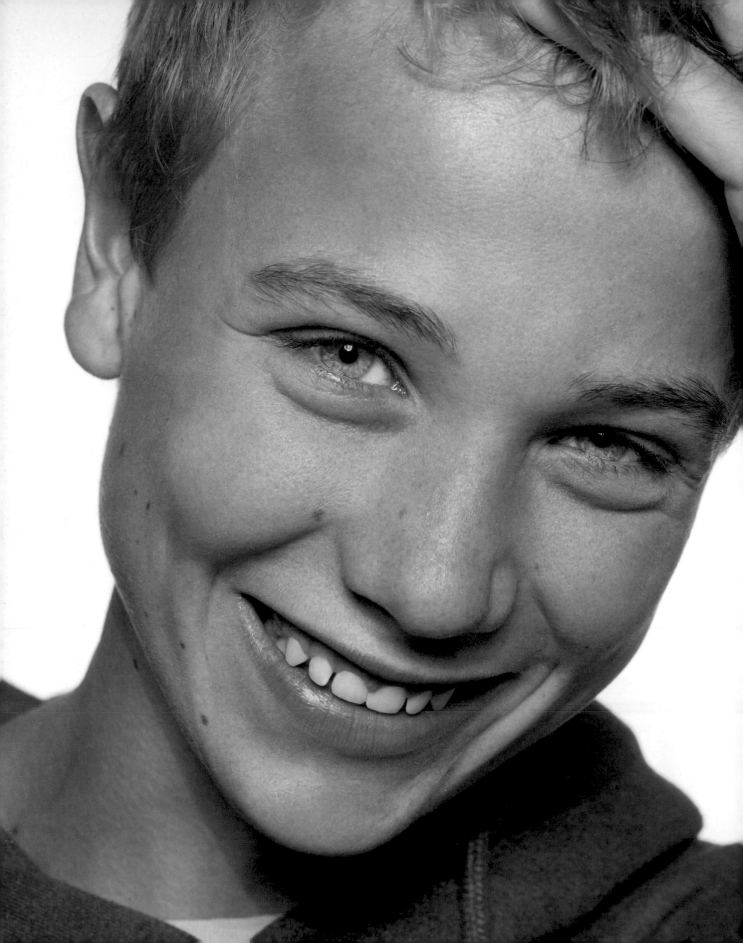

18

LET'S HEAR IT FOR THE BOYS

Guys like to pretend they don't care about how they look. Sure, there are those who spend more time on their hair than I do and are on a first-name basis with the salesperson at the men's products department-store counter. But being a mother and aunt of so many of them, I can tell you boys usually don't ask beauty questions. Or grooming questions. Or hygiene questions. Or fashion questions.

Caring about your appearance is not just for girls. It's important that boys know how to shave the right way—by lathering up the area with a bar of soap (rather than shaving cream) to soften the hair follicles so they don't get a rash and ingrowns. They also need to pay attention to cutting their nails. There's nothing worse than looking at a cute guy and seeing he has awful nails. Those things do matter. And why are boys so afraid of lotion?

If you have a boyfriend, brother, or best friend who could use a little help with his routine, my advice is to nudge him gently. Don't nag. Offer these tips in a cool, laid-back way. And if he takes your advice, follow it up by telling him how good he looks. That gets them every time.

gross habit:

He shaves his face like he's clearing a forest. He's so rough with the razor that angry red bumps rise up almost immediately when he's done.

groomed solution:

The first mistake most guys make is using the same razor for months (yuck). The razor blade should be changed after five to seven uses, or when the blade begins to pull on the skin. The shower—with shaving cream or soap, please!—is the best place for shaving because the steam opens up the pores and plumps the hair. This makes for a smoother shave and reduces the chances of nicks. He shouldn't forget to check his work. You can buy him a fog-free mirror that works in a steamy place to avoid the dreaded patch of hair left after a shave. Buy him aftershave or face cream specially designed to soothe the face after a shave. This will help a lot with razor burn and smells nice. If you are having a hard time convincing him of the benefits of a shave done right, take him to a pro. Once he feels his smooth face after the work of hot steam and a sharp razor, he won't go back to his brutal ways.

gross habit:

He uses harsh bar soap to wash his face. The formula and heavy deodorants in those soaps, created to fight the heaviest dirt and grime, strip skin of necessary oils. They leave his skin so tight he can hardly crack a smile.

groomed solution:

Offer him a lathering cleanser that's specially created for the face but has the same suds as his old bar of soap. Put it in the shower for him; otherwise, trust me, he'll never use it.

gross habit:

He's got an out-of-control unibrow.

groomed solution:

Nobody likes a unibrow, not even guys. Get a pair of sturdy tweezers into his hands and tell him to pluck only the hairs in-between his brows (believe it or not, boys can over-tweeze, too). Make sure the tweezers have a flat slanted edge, not pointed, for easier plucking.

gross habit:

He's had the same haircut since he was seven years old.

groomed solution:

It's hard to wean guys away from the corner barber, who shears their hair like they are a bunch of sheep. And just when it's grown in and looking cute again, they head right back to that barber chair. Try luring your guy to a salon. If yours is too over-the-top or feminine, find a cool, low-key place that has a lot of male clients. At first he might be embarrassed, but the luxury of having his hair washed will surely win him over. Just make sure the salon isn't super-pricey. There's nothing guys like to spend less on than hair.

gross habit:

His feet smell so bad that when he takes his shoes off, you almost pass out.

groomed solution:

Smelly feet come from sweat, which creates bacteria with bad odors. Feet get sweaty when guys are active or wear thick sports socks or shoes in materials that don't breathe. Not wearing socks with shoes and wearing the same pair of shoes every day are two big culprits behind stinky feet. Encourage him to put away his favorite sneaks for a day and rotate his shoes. Putting powder in sneakers and shoes is also a good way to absorb odor. Every once in a while, he should wash his sneakers with cold water (don't put them in the dryer, or they'll shrink). Some dry-cleaners also have sneaker cleaners. If the bad foot smell persists, he should see a doctor because some foot odors are caused by a fungus that needs to be treated with prescription medicine.

gross habit:

His idea of moisturizing his lips is to lick them when they are dry.

groomed solution:

Spit is not a product, OK? Licking your lips actually dries them out. When saliva evaporates, it strips the lips' natural oils, leaving them even more chapped. Buy your guy a clear, unscented lip balm that's small enough for him to stick in his jeans pocket.

gross habit:

He gets pimples on his chest and back that he loves to make a hobby out of picking.

groomed solution:

Although it's tempting, picking often leads to infection and sometimes, even worse, scarring. The best way to keep him from picking is to keep the pimples from arising in the first place. Have him try a body wash with salicylic acid, which gets rid of the dead skin cells that clog pores and cause pimples.

gross habit:

He's really careless about his sunscreen. At the beach, he slaps a palm or two of sunblock on his back and cheeks so that at the end of the day, he looks like a patchwork quilt of color.

groomed solution:

For beach days or outdoor sports, get him a spray-on waterproof sunscreen. The spray formula is easy to apply. Add a daily face moisturizer with sunscreen to protect against the majority of UVA and UVB exposure that he'll get.

gross habit:

He bites his nails until they are a jagged mess.

groomed solution:

Try treating him to a real manicure. I'm not talking red polish here. Lots of men get manicures at salons—hold the polish. If he has neatly trimmed nails, there won't be anything to bite. Plus, he'll love the feeling of the hand massage that usually comes with the manicure.

gross habit:

His locker smells like something died in it.

groomed solution:

Check to see if it's last year's tuna sandwich causing the smell. Then get him some fabric softener sheets to put in his locker, or a box of baking soda. Both will absorb odors (the fabric conditioner has the bonus of a scent that can mask almost anything).

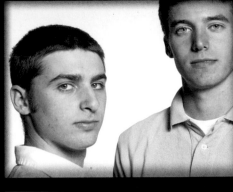
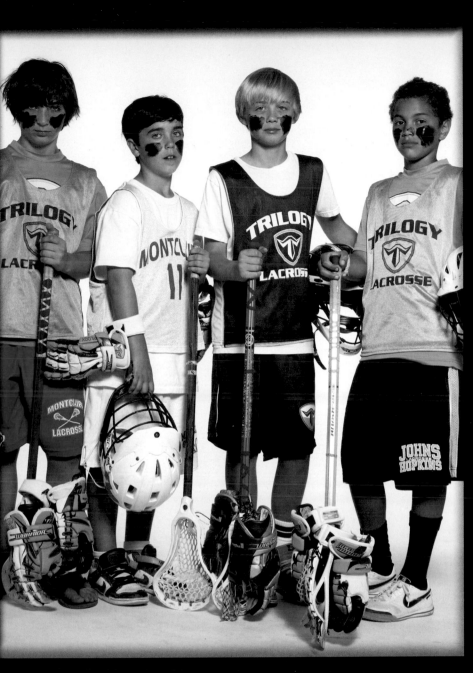
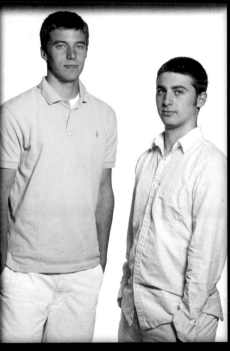
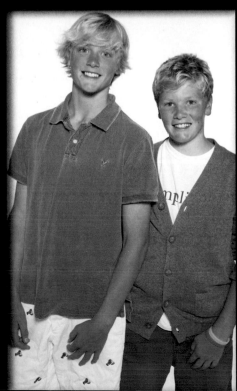
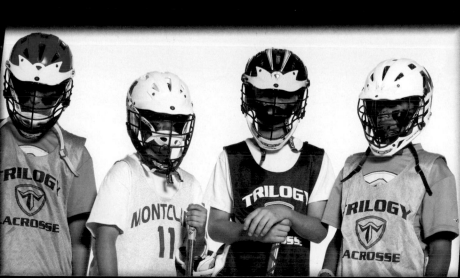

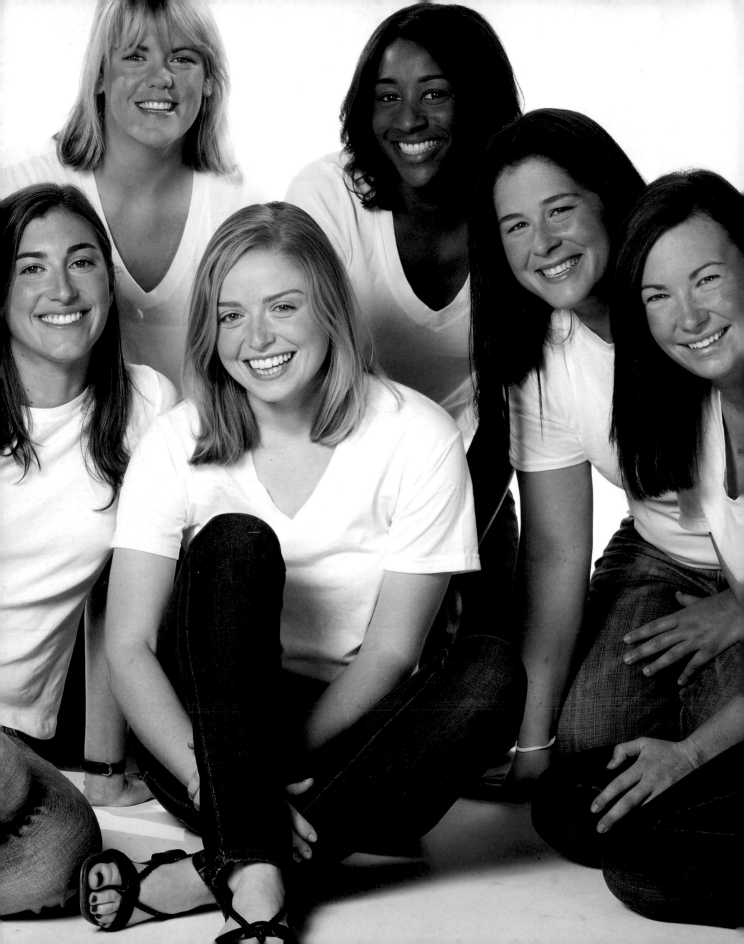

19

TEN YEARS LATER

It is pretty astounding how fast ten years goes by. I have watched with amazement how the girls who were in my first teen book ten years ago have grown into women. They have transformed from insecure kids, unsure of themselves in this confusing world, to vibrant, smart young women ready to take on the world.

Girls these days are much more sophisticated than they were when I wrote my first book (who thought it was possible?). There is so much more information out there on the Internet, on TV, and in magazines. It's practically impossible to be naive about anything, from fashion to politics. The modern media blitz means a lot more negative images populating the minds of young people. But there are just as many incredible role models staking their claim on this society. Rather than concerning themselves about the latest "it" bag, I think girls these days are inspired by do-gooders such as Bono, who's devoted to raising money and awareness for Africa; Oprah, who has helped all of us better ourselves for years; or Barack and Michelle Obama, who are all about helping people help themselves.

Young people are on the forefront of some of today's biggest issues, including the environment, education, and global poverty. But to do good things in the world, you have to feel good about yourself. That's why I wanted the girls from the original book—who made it through their teen years and lived to tell about it—to talk about their experiences now that they have some perspective. All the ups and downs of being a girl are really normal, even if you don't realize it at the time. Hearing about someone who's been there before, and come through the other end, is very empowering. Just like the girls ten years ago, you are okay now, and you will be okay in the future.

kate

twenty-two, just graduated from Amherst College and is hoping to become a social worker.

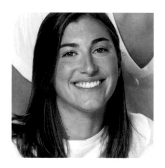

THEN: A lot in my life was changing. I was making new friends, realizing that there was more music out there than the Spice Girls and the Beatles, and really developing my own sense of style and personality. . . . I was even more of a tomboy then than I am now, so my lack of style back then makes me cringe. I liked baggy straight-leg pants to the point of almost buying the same as my brother. And my eyebrows—let's just say I get them from my dad.

NOW: I'm interested in the way people think and interact. I hope to do social work with youth and am concerned about the need for all children to grow up in healthy, supportive environments. In college, I loved being on our track team. During the past two summers, I've led bike trips in Vermont and on the Pacific Coast. I absolutely loved that free-spirited, outdoor-adventure experience. . . . What I've learned since I was a teen is that it's always okay to just be yourself. Who you're friends with will naturally change over the course of your life, and soon enough you'll find yourself surrounded by people who want you to be you and appreciate everything you are.

meg

twenty-two, just graduated from Colgate University.

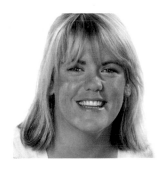

THEN: I was really obsessed with sports at the time—both soccer and softball. I also had a really great group of friends at my middle school, and we were kind of obsessed with each other. I also had an obsession with Jennifer Aniston—I wanted to be her! This is so cheesy, but I remember that when the book came out, I was so pumped that there was a picture of her in it so I could say that I was in a book with her! I loved Hollywood and celebrities. . . . I also used to wear my hair really, really tightly pulled back with this horrendous bun in the back, and then I would pull two pieces of hair out so that there was one on either side of my face. I remember thinking it was so awesome, but it was definitely not. I always wore oversize T-shirts with jeans, tucking the front in and leaving the back out. I thought I looked smaller by wearing big clothes, but I'm pretty sure it had the opposite effect.

NOW: I'm still obsessed with sports. Softball and soccer have defined so much of who I am and what I've chosen to do. When I studied abroad in England my junior year, I joined a soccer team and was able to make friends with so many people. I love that amazing quality about sports teams, the way they have connected me with people I may never have known and have brought me so many opportunities (like being in a Bobbi Brown book). I'm at a huge turning point in my life. Having just graduated, I'm trying to figure out where I want to go and what I want to be. Although it's kind of scary, it's also really exciting to have so much choice and freedom to be whatever I'd like. I'm excited to see where the next few years will take me.

rebecca h.

twenty-two, is a research economist and contributing editor at the Economic Cycle Research Institute.

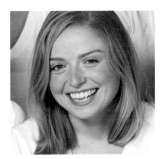

THEN: At twelve years old, I read and played soccer incessantly and tried anything I could to be different from my older sister. . . . I was really shy growing up, but I learned that getting out of your element—taking random classes, spending time with different people, going new places—is the best way to figure out who you want to be. You're potentially capable of living very different lives. The trick is to find out which one is most satisfying.

NOW: These days I love to write—travel writing and economic research are my passion and intellectual challenge. And I still play soccer in New York City.

julianne

twenty-two, attends graduate school at James Madison University.

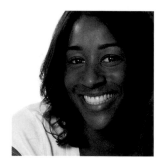

THEN: When I think back to middle school, I mostly laugh because I went through a different phase every year. One year I spent trying to be really girly and dress up for school regularly. The next year I was trying to be punk or emo and had three fake pairs of leather pants that I would wear at least once a week. I don't think I would ever wear pleather again . . . . I remember learning from Bobbi how to make my makeup look subtle but beautiful. The trick was to put it on and still look natural. Back then my favorite Bobbi Brown item was the lip gloss. There was a color that looked perfect on me, and I wore it every day until I lost it.

NOW: I received my undergrad degree, and now I am doing one more year to get my master's so I can teach elementary school. Right now I am very passionate about becoming a teacher. I plan to get a job in Virginia teaching or possibly leave the country and go to South America and teach there for a year or two. I keep my future in mind with everything I do.

chloe c.

twenty-two, is in her final year at Clark University, where she plays for the basketball team.

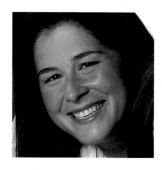

THEN: I wish that as a teen I had been more aware that it is okay to just be yourself. Realizing that I was gay at a young age was a battle because nobody else around me seemed to be going through the same thing. I wish I had known that it was okay because that is who I am and it doesn't matter how people around you act or what they feel; you will truly find yourself much happier, more confident, and comfortable when you find yourself and embrace it because it is you.

NOW: My biggest passion is basketball. I love to play it, watch it, coach it—just be involved with it on any level. I am concerned with our environment, civil rights, and mostly making the world a better place.

molly

twenty-two, is getting a master's degree in elementary education.

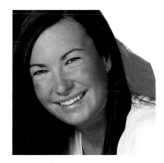

THEN: I was just making the change from tomboy to dressing girly, and I started mimicking all the seventh-grade girl trends of the time. There are definitely some things that stand out in my mind as fashion don'ts that I did a lot of. For example, glittery butterfly clips all over my head, eye shadow up past my eyebrows in purples and blues, and the braided and beaded hairdo that every girl begged for on vacation.

NOW: Obviously, a lot changes between the ages of twelve and twenty-two. I now know that makeup is really fun and useful when you know how to use it but that you have to be confident with yourself first to pull it off. I'm also passionate about school and education in general. I love kids, which has driven me to become a teacher. I understand and care a lot more about the world around me than I did ten years ago. I'm still really close with my friends, and I don't think that will ever change.

lindsay

thirty-two, is a senior writer at *ESPN The Magazine.*

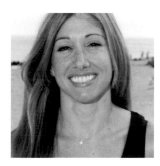

THEN: I was obsessed with getting my foot in the door as a sportswriter. I played soccer, ice hockey, and softball growing up and through college. I've been an athlete my whole life, and working out in the morning helps me concentrate on what I need to do with the rest of my day. I used to also spend a lot more time on my hair and makeup back then.

NOW: I'm lucky, I really love my job. I love the writing, I love the opportunity it affords me to travel all over the world covering sporting events, and I love all the people I meet along the way. Now, I don't have to blow-dry my hair all the time. I don't mind throwing it up wet into a bun, and I don't really wear a full face of makeup unless I'm going out. Just tinted moisturizer, mascara, and lip balm for me now. I wish somebody had told me when I was younger that zits do not stop when you turn twenty-one, or twenty-five, or thirty. If they're typical for your skin type, you're going to get them. And they're not the end of the world, because nine times out of ten, nobody notices them but you.

chloe s.

twenty-one, works at Polo Ralph Lauren as an assistant to the senior vice president and vice president of design of Double RL.

THEN: I was obsessed with my friends and was just starting to get into makeup. I told everyone I was going to be a makeup artist. I remember wanting to be just like Bobbi. I was so young, but those middle-school years were when my friends and I really started to care about our appearance, how boys perceived us, what clothes we liked. . . . I will never forget doing the book—it was such a great experience. I must admit I was a little shy about being in the braces chapter. Of course, when you are that age and your metal mouth is highlighted it is embarrassing, but now it is very funny to look back on . . . I mean, really funny!

NOW: Now that I am in my early twenties, I feel much more comfortable, I know exactly what I like and don't like—there is no more "figuring it out." I am sure of my style, what products I like, what shades to wear, how I do my makeup and hair, and what looks good on my body. It all just comes naturally now, whereas when I was a young teen, I was constantly trying things out because I wasn't sure what worked for me. . . . I just graduated from the University of San Diego, and now I am reestablishing myself back on the East Coast with a new job and apartment in Manhattan with my best friend. The most important thing to me now is succeeding in work and keeping close with my family. My parents and I have a friendship that's too good to be true, and as I've grown up, I have realized that not everyone is so lucky.

jessica

twenty-four, jewelry designer.

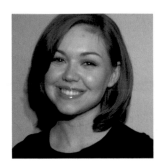

THEN: I was probably mostly into boys. I had braces and was kind of awkward. I spent a lot of time making art and dreaming about my future. I would wear anything weird and different that I could get my hands on. I needed to be different.

NOW: I'm still into clothes and fashion. I'm also passionate about working with my hands, being artistic by making jewelry, sketching, and writing. I also love to cook. Learning to cook really opened my eyes to all the amazing food out there. I took my teen years too seriously. I always held back a lot. Just have fun!

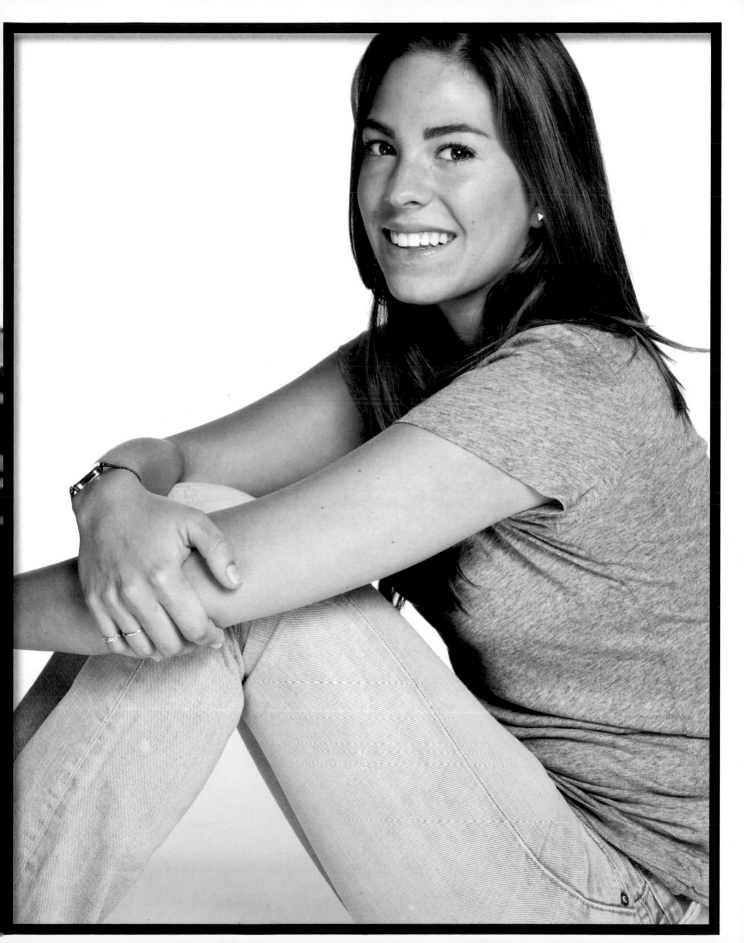

THESE GIRLS SURVIVED THEIR TEENS.

YOU WILL TOO.

nefertiti

twenty-three, is a student at the University of Pittsburgh.

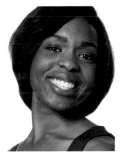

THEN: At the time of the book, I ate, slept, and drank dance. I used to wear my hair out in this huge semi-fro. I say it was a *semi*-fro because my hair was relaxed, but I just tweezed it a little bit. After I spent an hour working in front of the mirror, my hair would go from flat to a huge puff. I loved it. I just can't believe I spent a ridiculous amount of time trying to perfect that style. . . . The biggest thing I learned from Bobbi Brown's book ten years ago is that less is more. Your face doesn't have to be saturated in makeup for you to look stunning. Instead, a dab of makeup here and there can take you a long way!

NOW: Dance continues to be my passion. During my time at the University of Pittsburgh, I performed in many plays through a performing group named Kuntu Repertory. One thing I've learned in the last ten years is that you can't please everyone, so stop trying! Focus on pleasing yourself, and that will take you very far in life.

chloe k.

twenty-three, just graduated from Boston University and hopes to get a job that relates to psychology or social work before she returns to graduate school.

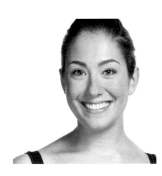

THEN: I was a very, very small girl and obsessed with growing. All of my peers were developing, and I hadn't even begun. I really wanted to fit in. I prayed every night to grow, especially for breasts. Little did I know a year or so later they would be bigger than every single one of my friends' breasts. I think I might have prayed too hard, hence, my current double-D breasts. I was also obsessed with dancing, which was my way of expressing myself and relieving my stress. I literally lived in my leotard and tights at the time! . . . I also was really set on being perfect, or what I thought perfection was. I have now accepted that there is no such thing as perfection and to love myself just the way I am, flaws and all.

NOW: I want to make sure I find a job that I enjoy and make sure that my skills in psychology are being utilized. Another concern of mine is that because I have stopped dancing, I need to find another form of physical exercise to keep me healthy in both body and mind. I have tried yoga and even had a personal trainer for a while, but I have not found an activity that gives me that same wonderful feeling that dance did. I might just have to sign up for a few dance classes and try to get back into it!

gretchen

twenty-seven, works in public relations for Bobbi Brown Cosmetics.

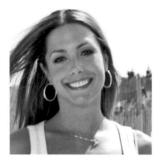

THEN: I was obsessed with school, sports, friends, boys, makeup, and talking on the phone. I also remember I used to match my eye shadow to the color of the clothes I was wearing. For my junior prom, I had a green iridescent dress with eye shadow to match. Awful!

NOW: It's all about my fiancé, family, friends, work, reading, and traveling. I've also learned you need to have confidence in yourself. That is the foundation for looking and feeling your best.

rebecca p.

twenty-six, is senior manager of development and events at Endeavor, an economic development nonprofit company.

THEN: Ten years ago, my aunt Bobbi hosted my sweet-sixteen birthday party for a group of my friends. She offered us a simple, but empowering message that I still find applicable today—you are young; enhance your natural beauty; drink lots of water; get sleep; and remember that you look your best when you are happy.

NOW: Nobody says that the teenage years are easy. Despite all the advice I ever received, I've become the person I am today by making my own mistakes. From falling in love to getting my heart broken to worrying about weight to graduating to living on my own—these experiences define who I am. The reality is that you never stop caring about what others think of you. But if you are confident and can stand by your decisions, then you are on the right path.

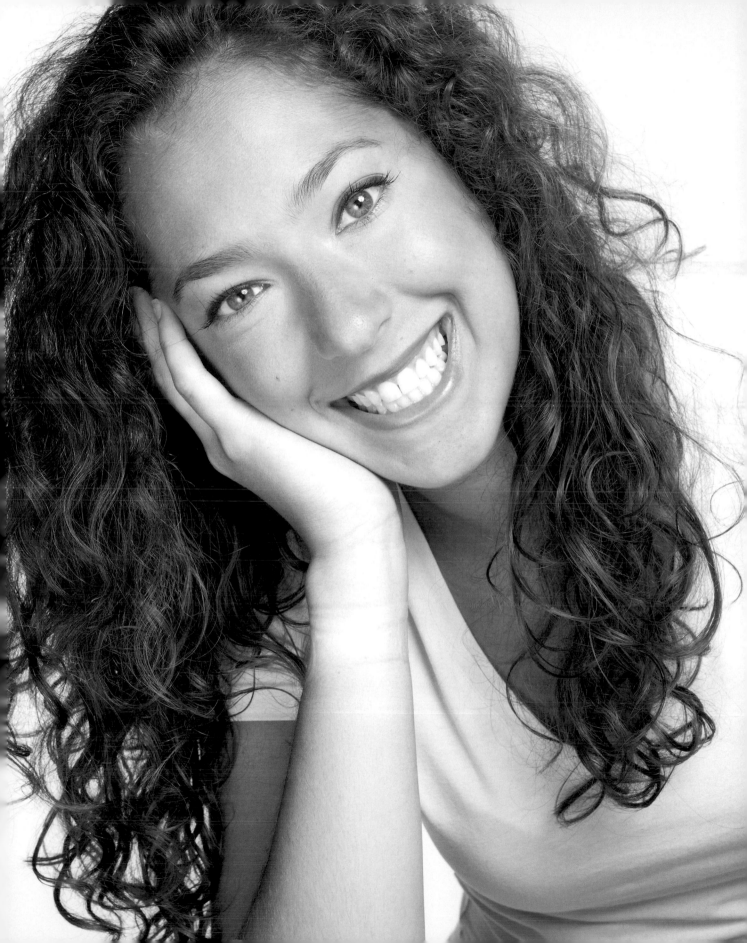

ACKNOWLEDGMENTS

SPECIAL ACKNOWLEDGMENTS

JILL COHEN for putting and keeping this project together

REBECCA PALEY for perfectly simple and funny words

ONDREA BARBE for amazing and stunning photos and being so grounded

CHRISTINE CARSWELL for constant support, enthusiasm, and vision

SARA SCHNEIDER for being open and finding our groove

KATE WOODROW for your fabulous editorial input

TERA KILLIP for getting the printing perfect

KIM COLVILLE for being the glue and diving right in

TORI SMYLY for keeping me sane (and awesome protein shakes)

BEN RITTER for being so cool and taking the best photos effortlessly

TZVETA STAMATOVA for perfection

ERIC DOMINGUEZ for being calm and precise

MAUREEN CASE for just being you

GENERAL ACKNOWLEDGMENTS

MAKEUP ARTISTS
KIMBERLY CHRISTINE SOANE
WALTAYA CULMER
CASSANDRA GARCIA
RICKI GURTMAN
KIM HARRISON
TIA HEBRON
JOHN HERNANDEZ
ELIZABETH KEISER
DOMINIQUE NAMOLI
MARC REAGAN
SASHA GROSSMAN, ASSISTANT

BOBBI BROWN PUBLIC RELATIONS TEAM
VERONIKA ULLMER
ALEXIS RODRIGUEZ
CECILE ABEILLE
CLAIRE GOODWIN
GRETCHEN BERRA
ELIZABETH JUST
SAMANTHA BAILYE
JOAN JUENGLING

PHOTOGRAPHY
IAN GIPE—
    AGENT TO ONDREA BARBE
JOE LEONARD—
    SECOND ASSISTANT
JUSTIN FRANCAVILLA—
    FIRST ASSISTANT
ALEX YERKS—
    DIGITAL TECHNICIAN
BRAD JAMIESON—
    SHOOT DIGITAL

FILM/VIDEO PRODUCTION
ELLEN LEWIS
VICTORIA KRESS
ETHAN MASS—
    CAMERA
STU WEINBERG—
    AUDIO

THE BOBBI BROWN STUDIO, MONTCLAIR NEW JERSEY
THANK YOU FOR ALWAYS BEING THERE,
    DOORS OPEN.
KIM HARRISON
WALTAYA CULMER
BRIELLE OLIASTRO
DOMINIQUE NAIMOLI
EMILY MCHUGH

SHOOT PRODUCTION
LINDSEY JACKSON—
    PRODUCTION ASSISTANT
CIERRA SHERWIN—
    PRODUCTION ASSISTANT
ERIC DOMINGUEZ—
    HAIR
KIM HOWARD—
    HAIR ASSISTANT
ROZA ISRAEL—
    MANICURIST
RALPH IZZARD—
    STUDIO MANAGER
RON HILL—
    DRIVER

CATERING
SESAME RESTAURANT
FALAFEL HUT
MARKET RESTAURANT
MISS NICKY
MARCIN MROZ

J. CREW
MICKEY DREXLER
JENNA LYONS
HEATHER MCAULIFFE
    AND THE REST OF THE J. CREW TEAM
MARISSA CRAWFORD—
    SHOOT STYLIST
LAUREN PRICE—
    SHOOT STYLING ASSISTANT
MADELINE GARBER—
    SHOOT STYLING ASSISTANT

BOBBI BROWN COSMETICS
ESPECIALLY
DAVID NASS
ANNEMARIE IVERSON
DOROTHY MANCUSO
RUBA ABU-NIMAH
KRISTEN BOSCAINO
JOHN EATON

ADDITIONAL SUPPORT
LARISA MAKOW
LPGA
CHURCH STREET OPTICIANS
ROBIN SCHLAGER
JONI BRONANDER
SCOTT AND PILAR KENNEDY
    AT ALPHAGRAPHICS

THANK YOU TO OUR MODELS

SYDNEY ABAJIAN, CHANELLE ADAMS, KRISTIE AHN, EMMA ALHALEL, HANNAH ALHALEL, JILLIAN ALONZO, GABRIELLE ALVES, NEFERTITI ALVES, GABBY AMBROSIO, ANA ANBAR, COBY ANTINORO, JACQUIE ANTINORO, REMI ANTINORO, SAMANTHA BAILYE, RACHEL BAKER, AURORA BAUMBACH, SAMANTHA BEDOL, LEXI BEECHLER, JACKIE BENDETH, LIA BENTLEY, ALEXANDRE BENYA, GRETCHEN BERRA, LINDSAY BERRA, KAILA BIGELOW, MAGGIE BIGELOW, MELISSA BIGELOW, SAVANNAH BIGELOW, JAYANNA BROWN, MARIAELENA BROWN, MARLENNE BROWN, TESSA CALANDRA, ALESSANDRA CANARIO, SABRINA CANARIO, SUSANA CANARIO, ANNA CARDELFE, CHLOE CARDIN, MOLLY CAREY, ELIZABETH COHEN, MARGARET COHEN, TAYLOR COHEN, HARRY COLVILLE, JAKE COLVILLE, BRITTANY COOPER, LISA COOPER, JUSTINE CRAWFORD, MARISSA CRAWFORD, ALEXANDRA CRUZ, MADISYN CULMER, WALTAYA CULMER, SARA DANA, KAT DELUNA, MIA DESIMONE, DIANNE DEWITT, GABI DOLCE-BENGTSSON, JESSICA DREWITZ, TYLER DREWITZ, DARA DUFFY, KELSEY DUFFY, SHANE DUFFY, AMELIA DUNNELL, KAITLYN EDA, KAREN NIKKO EDA, KAYLA EDA, EVE EGBERT, JAMES EVANS, OLIVIA EVANS, JACQUELYN FELICIANO, KATELYN FELICIANO, KRISTALYN FELICIANO, MICHEAUX FERDINAND, CLAIRE FITZGERALD, CHLOE FONT, DANIELA FUENTES, MADELINE GARBER, GENEVIEVE GEANEY, NANCY DEWEIR GEANEY, LAINIE GILBERT, SAM GILBERT, GRACE GILL, JANE GILL, JENNY GOLDSTEIN, KARINA GOMEZ, LOGAN GREENE, TAYLOR GREGORY, ROSEANNE GUARARRA, AMANDA HALTMAIER, HEATHER HAMMERLING, KYLA HANSEN, ELIZABETH HARNETT, KELLEY HARTMANN, MEG HEISLER, CLAIRE HENTSCHKER, KIM HOLLAND, DANIELLE HOLMAN, LALLY HOMANS, MARDET HOMANS, TYLER HONSINGER, REBECCA HOUSTON, EMILY JACKSON, HAYLEY JACKSON, JULIE JACKSON, LINDSEY JACKSON, ERINN JENKINS, KAILA JENKINS, PAM JENKINS, TIFFANY JENKINS, KAROLINA JEWETT, MARLENA JEWETT, SASHA JEWETT, KATE JOYCE, MOLLY JOYCE, JOAN JUENGLING, KC KAICHER, CHLOE KATZ, JUSTINE KAY, KATE KELLY, EMILY KLEIN, AVA KRAVITZ, AVIVA KUSHNER, HANNAH KUSHNER, DANI LAWRENCE-COHEN, YASMIN LEUTWYLER, ALEXANDRA TROWER LINDSEY, GRACE LINDSEY, JENNA LYONS, SHANNON MACAULAY, DANIELA MARTINEZ, MOLLY MCALVANAH, ALISON MCCLEARN, KATHY MCCLEARN, MARY GORMAN MCCOY, MOLLY MCCOY, REILLY MCCOY, KATE MCVEIGH, ADRIENNE MENICHESCHI, CHRISTOPHER MERCADO, JULIANNE MERRICK, JILLIAN MIZRAJI, NADIA MOREHAND, SIMA MORGELLO, SARAH MORRISSEY, SETA MORTON, MEG MYLAN, KATE O'CONNOR, SAM O'HARA, SCOUT OPATUT, BECCA PLOFKER, CODY PLOFKER, DUKE PLOFKER, DYLAN PLOFKER, KATYA POLIAKOFF, ATHIANA PORTILLO, MORGAN PRESSEL, MANDA GARCIA PYSZCZYMUKA, NOELLE RASCO, LENA RAWLEY, KIARA ROBERSON, STEPHANIE ROMBOUGH, MELINDA ROY, OLIVIA SAGE-EL, ALEXIS SARANDON, LISA SARANDON, KELLY SARANDON, STEPHANIE SARANDON, ANDIE SCHER, HANNA SCHLAGER, SARAH SCHMIDT, NICOLE SCOTT, AMANDA SEAMAN, MELISSA SEEPERSAND, SARAH SHERMAN, SUNNY SHOKRAE, SHONTELLE, ALICE SHORTALL, AMANDA SHORTALL, CHLOE SILBER, CHARLOTTE SILVERMAN, DREW SILVERMAN, KATE SILVERMAN, CHRISTINA SILWAK, NOLAN SMITH, PAIGE SMITH, SARAYA SMITH, ELIZABETH STARNES, KIMBERLY STRATTON, SAVANNAH STRENZ, LILY SUSMAN, LISA SWENSON, LAUREN THOMAS, LYNN THOMAS, GENEVIEVE VAN LENT, MARIELLE VERNI , MICHELLE WARANADE, HIILLARY WELDON, WHITNEY WELDON, MELISSA WREDE, MIMI WREDE, WILL WREDE, AND KORINNA WRIGHT

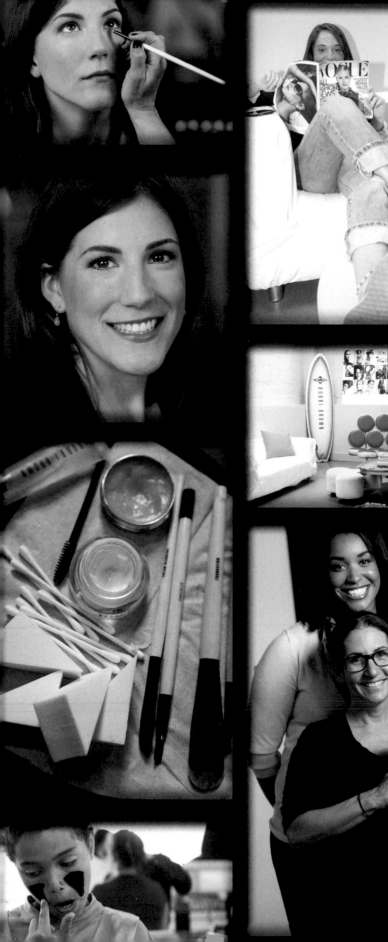
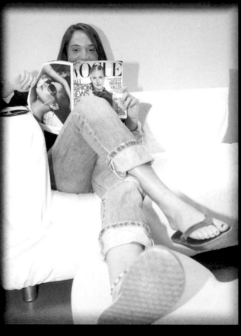
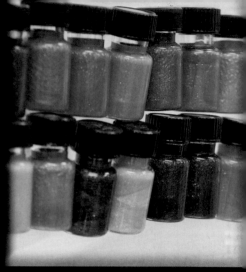
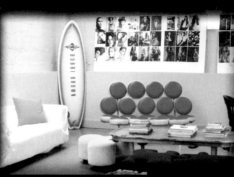
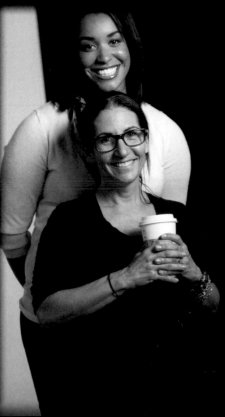
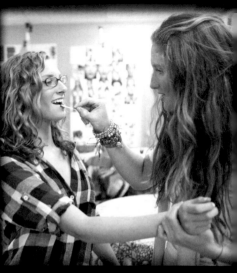
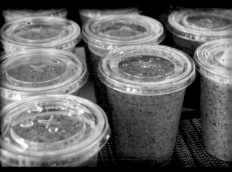
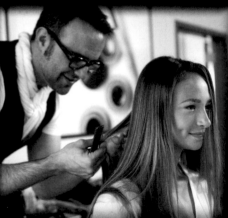

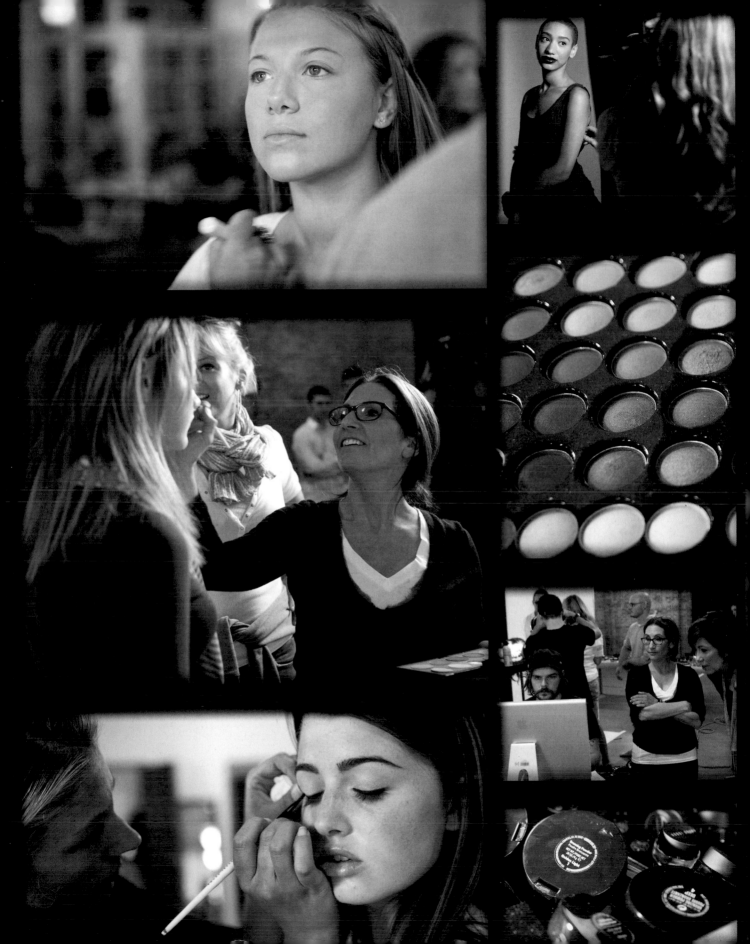

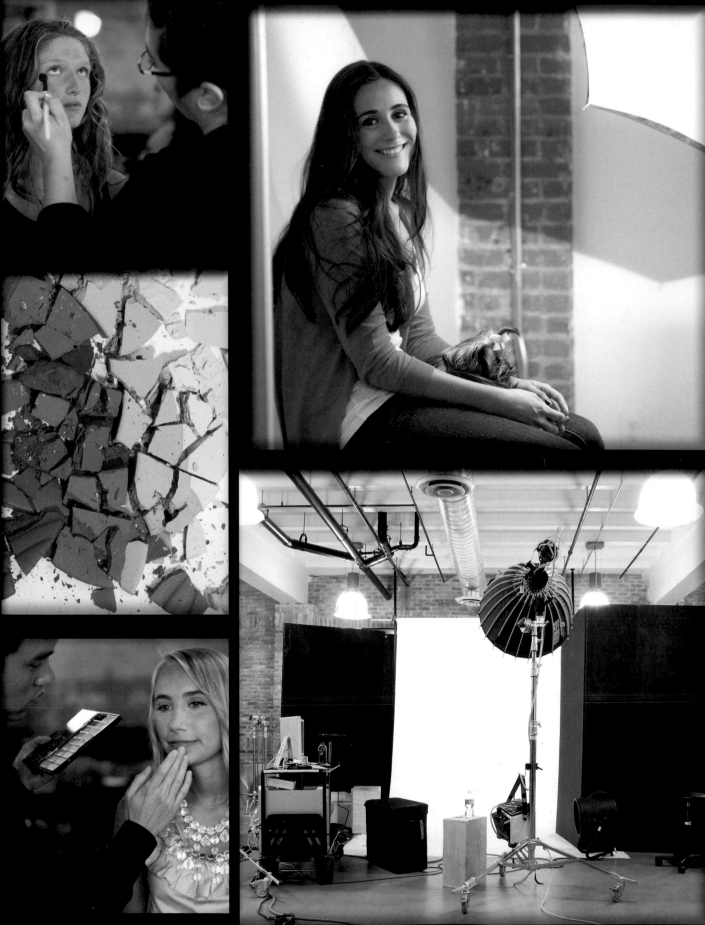

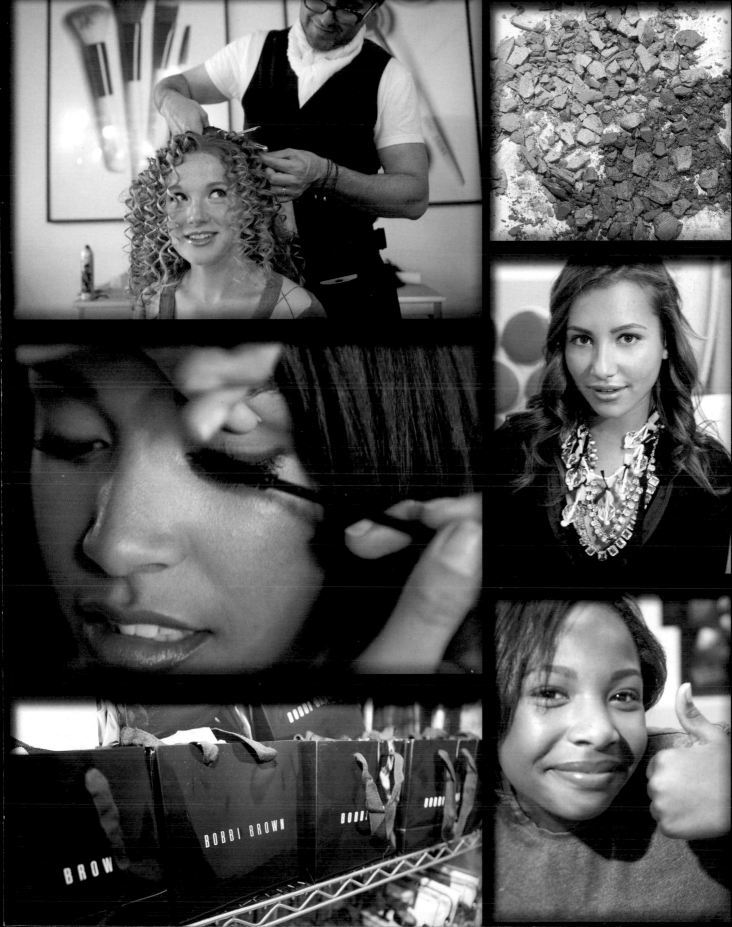

INDEX

DON'T FORGET THE LAST BEAUTY RULE . . .

RULES
ARE MADE TO BE
BROKEN

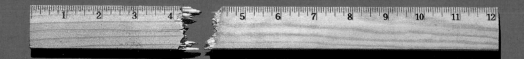